Nursing and the American Health Care Delivery System

Nursing and the American Health Care Delivery System

Fourth Edition

Joellen W. Hawkins, R.N.C., Ph.D., F.A.A.N.
Professor, Boston College

Loretta P. Higgins, R.N., Ed.D.
Associate Professor and Associate Dean, Boston College

The Tiresias Press, Inc., New York City

To our families, friends, colleagues, and students.

Preface

This book on the health care delivery system is intended as a text for undergraduate and graduate nursing students. Beginning with concepts from general systems theory, it examines various facets of health care delivery in the United States. Woven throughout are the historical threads that form the fabric of today's system. The impact of the multiplicity of public and private providers who are responsible for health care and the influence of various power groups on health care delivery are discussed. The effect of legislation on health care provision and on nursing practice is emphasized. The book explores health-related industries, the cost of health care and who pays, the role of consumers, and barriers to care experienced by certain groups. A brief exploration of the selected systems in other countries is followed by projections for the future and a discussion of current trends in health care. Throughout the book, the roles of nurses and nursing are emphasized.

To students preparing to enter the health care delivery system as providers and potential change agents, an understanding of how the present so-called system functions, and its strengths and weaknesses, would seem imperative to professional practice. It is our hope that this book will served as an introduction to and exploration of the ways in which health and illness care are delivered in the United States and of plans for changes.

Acknowledgements

The authors wish to express their gratitude to their colleagues and especially to their students for assistance with this and each previous edition. This book is the product of needs expressed by students for a resource on the health care system focused on nurses and nursing. It developed out of a course on the health care system which we both taught.

We thank the many people who sent us materials on federal and state agencies, assisted us in library searches, and helped us to track down information.

Most of all, our thanks go to our ever-patient families and friends who continue to support and love us through project after project.

Contents

1

Applying General Systems Theory to Health Care Delivery

The roots of general systems theory (the concept that a system is the whole of its component parts) can be traced back centuries. A formal general systems theory was proposed by von Bertalanffy both in the 1930s and in his later publications (1; 2, p. 153). Boulding (3, p. 37) defined general systems theory as "a general science of wholeness." What is increasing in influence since the mid-forties is the *use* of general systems theory, which now stresses analysis of the whole as well as of the parts (4, p. 1). Even more recent is its application to health. General systems theory has important implications for use in organizing and analyzing our health care delivery system and its many subsystems. Furthermore, its application to the field of health research is important in providing a sound rationale for change.

We do not mean to suggest that general systems theory is the only way of looking at society or a segment of it. It is one method, however, that may be used to improve the public's satisfaction with the functioning of the health care system.

This country has birthed an amorphous giant known collectively as the health care delivery system. In reality, we know that system to be a collection of subsystems that are ill-matched, overlapping, full of gaps, and covered with Band-

Aids. A basic knowledge of general systems theory is of benefit to all health care providers in attempting both to understand (assess) our health care system and to change (intervene in) it. To that end, this chapter presents a summary of some of the basic concepts and terminology of general systems theory. Its application to the health care delivery system as a whole and to nursing in particular will then be discussed.

Basic Concepts

There are numerous definitions of the word "system." All of them, however, more or less agree that a system is a set of units or elements that actively interrelate and that may somehow be categorized as a unit (4, p. 5). Von Bertalanffy defines system as "a set of elements standing in interrelation among themselves and with the environment" (2, p.159). A system may be even more generally defined as a "purposeful collection of interacting entities"(5, p. 8). Boulding defines systems as "sets of elements standing in interaction" (3, p. 38). Thus, it becomes immediately apparent that a component of one system may also be a component of another. For example, a nurse may be a member of the subsystem of providers in the health care delivery system and, at the same time, be a member of a family system. From this illustration, it is obvious that one must take care in defining the system about which one is speaking or writing, unless the structure of the system is apparent to all. In referring to the health care delivery system in the United States, one may be referring to the entire conglomerate of private and public sectors with their providers, related industries, and services. Or one might be referring only to the institutions and persons, both private and public, that provide direct service to clients.

A number of classification levels for systems are found in the literature. One of the best known is that of Boulding (3, pp. 11-17), who lists the following: static (anatomy of the universe); simple dynamic (clockworks); cybernetic (level of a thermostat); open (the cell); genetic-societal (differentiation of cell labor);

animal (increased mobility, self-awareness); human (the individual); social (complexity of groups of individuals); and transcendental (ultimates and absolutes). Miller (6) describes the classical hierarchical levels of living systems moving from particles to atoms all the way up to ecological systems. He cites planets, solar systems, and galaxies as an example of levels into which a system might be classified. One of the classic writers in the field of systems theory, von Bertalanffy, (1) describes levels of systems as basic to organization in the biological world.

Terminology

The following systems terminology is adapted from Hazzard (7):

System: A set of interactional parts; a whole and its component parts. In health care delivery, the private and public institutions, individuals, goods, and services which are involved directly or indirectly in delivering health care to people (clients), or which are involved with people's physical and emotional well-being.

Subsystems: Those components of a system which may themselves be classified as systems. The institution we know as a hospital is one such example. The whole body of registered nurses in this country is another.

Suprasystem: The next highest system of which a given system is a component. Our United States health care delivery system might be viewed as a suprasystem, as could the conglomerate of health care systems of all the countries of the world.

Environment: Includes all the factors that influence and are affected by a system. The environment for health care in the United States is, in essence, the whole of the inhabited country with its geographic, economic, and political components, since each of these components influences and/or is influenced by the health care delivery system.

Closed System: One which has no interaction or interdependence with the environment. Actually, a system can only be relatively and never completely closed, although some say our health care delivery system for most of the 20th century has been closed, with the physician as gatekeeper. Some reformers of the present system want to make ours a much more open system.

Steady State: Adaptation of the system to change in order to maintain relative equilibrium. Each system has some tolerance for change. The United States' health care system adopted Medicare and Medicaid but managed to maintain relative equilibrium. There are those who believe that adoption of a national health insurance plan or some form of a national health scheme would upset the steady state.

Inputs: Elements taken into a system and transformed into outputs. The most obvious example in health care is its clients.

Outputs: Products of the system. In health care, outputs generally are healthier individuals or new human beings. The health care system also deals with entropy; the output then might be death with dignity.

Processor: Mechanisms that transform inputs to outputs. In health care, providers are processors, as are the technological devices and therapies they may use.

Transformation: The throughput processes which in some way change input to output. These may be human services, e.g., nursing care, medical care, medication, radiology, surgery, and so on.

Entropy: Breakdown; disorganization and disequilibrium; a measure of disorder in the system. A strike of health care workers in an institution may lead the system to entropy. Entropy for an individual is death.

Negentropy: Energy that can be used by the system; a measure of order or organization. The resources of a nursing staff available to the system is an example.

Feedback: Information on outputs and the condition of the operating systems. In our complex health care system, feedback on the nursing care we provide may be limited; we may never hear from a client again after he or she leaves the system. Recently, however, many institutions have initiated a system of eliciting feedback from clients by using questionnaires which clients complete as they are leaving the hospital.

Feedback Loop (Cybernetic Loop): The channels and directions in which feedback moves. Feedback from clients may help us to improve care; feedback from peers and supervisors may help us to change behavior and increase our accountability (8).

Morphogenesis: Refers to exchanges between the system and the environment that tend to alter the system in some way. For example, Congress may pass legislation that directly impacts on the health care delivery system, as when it passed Medicare and Medicaid bills in the 1960s.

Morphostasis: Processes that tend to preserve or maintain the form, structure, or state of a system. The lobbying activities of the American Medical Association might be an example.

Differentiation: Specialization within the system. This is very apparent in the plethora of specialists among physicians; there are also more than 400 subspecializations among providers within our health care delivery system.

Integration: Return to a less diffuse state. Coordination of care when a client is served by a variety of health care providers is one example of integration. Other examples are care by a primary care provider or a return by physicians to family practice.

Equifinality: Ability to reach a final state by a number of paths. A pertinent example is the several educational programs (diploma, associate degree, baccalaureate, masters, and doctoral) leading to qualifications for sitting for licensure examinations as a registered nurse.

Equicausality: The same cause may produce a variety of results under differing conditions. For one individual, aspirin may relieve pain; for another, it may cause severe bleeding; and for yet another, it may reduce inflammation.

Boundary Control: Refers to activities that preserve the boundaries of the system. Licensing examinations for professional nursing practice is one example; fees for membership in an HMO (health maintenance organization) is another.

Monitoring: Regulation of activity within a system. Nursing audit is one example; quality improvement programs is another.

Theoretical System: A paper exercise; an analytical system; a model. An example would be national health insurance plans under consideration in the early 1990s.

Real System: A concrete system, either humanly constructed or natural. The health care system is an example; a hospital is another.

Systems Analysis: Use of the problem-solving approach with the aid of technological advances such as computer systems and advanced business theories.

Application to the Health Care Delivery System

General systems theory is readily applicable to the health care delivery system as it presently exists in this country. Health care delivery is easily identifiable as a system or suprasystem with a vast number of systems or subsystems, including input (clients), throughput (health or illness care), and output (wellness or at least significant improvement in the majority of clients).

The health care delivery system, as we know it in this country, began with private physicians, healers, the religious, and midwives. The local community became involved to protect itself from the poor, the ill, and the insane — thus, the building of almshouses and asylums. Next, the federal government became involved, first with the well-being of its merchant seamen upon whom the colonies were so dependent, and then in assuming responsibility for the health screening of immigrants. Finally, in the nineteenth century, the states entered the health arena. Thus, we have a health care system which evolved from need rather than from a blueprint.

Until relatively recent times, this system has functioned more as an altruistic enterprise than as a business. It is now very much the latter. In fact, in terms of personpower, it is one of the biggest businesses in the country. Nearly 13% of our gross national product is spent on health care, and the industry employs over nine million persons (13).

Use of systems theory to describe the system and of systems analysis or the problem-solving approach can help us to unravel the complexity of so diverse a system as ours so that we can apply more effective means to control spiralling costs, improve output, reallocate resources, and fill the gaps so that equal access is a reality. The challenge, of course, is to retain humanistic qualities of caring in an age teeming with technology.

The systems approach has some distinct advantages to offer to our distraught health care system. "It is organized, creative, empirical, theoretical, and pragmatic" (5, p. 9). Like nursing process, it is based on the problem-solving approach and brings order to the processes of assessment, planning, implementation, and evaluation of situations in the real world of health care delivery. At the same time, it allows for the consideration of a number of creative alternative solutions and for planning based on past data such as utilization and costs. The ability to store and recall enormous amounts of data relating to a particular subsystem through integration of computer technology allows us to plan for projected, as well as for present, health care needs. For instance, knowing the facts about the utilization of health services by elderly citizens in a particular community over the past five years can help us to plan needed services on the basis of population, longevity, and available resources.

The large, complex United States health care system is not an organized system. Rather, it is a complexity of diverse systems, clumsily interacting with each other in random, often haphazard, modes (5, p. 31). The application of systems theory is an attempt to improve, or in some case to initiate, articulation. No longer can health care professionals afford to exist in their subsystems as if they were independent of environment and unrelated in any way to the rest of the system. Health care has become so complex that its two most traditional components, the solo medical practitioner and the community hospital, both of which have long operated largely on their own, have been forced to join the mainstream. Medicare, Medicaid, Blue Cross, Blue Shield, the more than 1,500 private insurance companies, HMOs, and other third-party payment plans have nudged and pushed these components into the twentieth century of big business health care, helped along by such bodies as the Joint Commission on Accreditation of Health Care Organizations (JCAHO) and a widespread call for health care reform from consumers and providers.

The underlying philosophy of this book is that the American health care system is not performing at the high level that is possible considering the available scientific and technological expertise and the monies that are spent on health-related activities. There are those who disagree. These people are satisfied with the present situation and insist that in this country one can find the highest level of health care in the world. They would hesitate to disrupt a system where such excellence has developed in an environment of free enterprise.

A number of objections to the systems approach to health care have been raised, the argument being that services to people can never be quantified, analyzed, and systematized. However, there is little to support retention of our present way of operating and much to suggest that new approaches are needed. The challenge is to find ways to utilize the best that our technology can offer while at the same time maintaining or returning to a people-oriented health care system available to all. There is hope in the statement of Miller who, in writing of the application of the general systems approach to clients, said, "As we extend our basic research in systems service we may well obtain new understanding which will enable us to improve our health care delivery system" (9, p. 83).

Application to Nursing

If nurses are to continue to gain credibility for the practice of nursing, we must develop power as members of the professional health care delivery team based on our expertise. And that expertise will come from theory and research in nursing. King urges the application of systems theory and systems research to the task of providing a sound theoretical and research foundation for nursing practice (10, pp. 51-60).

Each nursing situation encountered is very complex. Changes since the mid-nineteenth century, when nursing as a profession was in its infancy, have largely been technological and mechanical. The clients have changed little. As health care providers, we interact with individuals, families, groups, communities, and society. The expectations for nursing performance are much more complex than they were a century ago. Nurses must master a great deal of technological information, function in a variety of settings, assume management responsibilities in large and complex organizations, and synthesize learning from a variety of disciplines in which we take courses as part of our professional education. Every day nurses make countless observations of clients. Yet little is done with the data we collect (10, pp. 57-59).

Thus, systems theory can be utilized to help us order knowledge, analyze the components that comprise professional practice, and, most of all, use rather than discard the data we collect to strengthen the base for practice. Furthermore, the systems approach may be used to evaluate the quality of patient care (11). We have had little useful feedback to help us to support or alter modes of care delivery until recently. The systems model helps us to definite goals, identify variables, and measure the output of nursing service to clients. General systems theory can provide a theoretical framework for organizing nursing activities in relation to clients, families, and communities. For example, we deal with entropy, evaluation, and equifinality with clients (12).

The most attractive part of systems theory to the practice of professional nursing is its emphasis on the whole. Nursing purports to be concerned with the whole human being as client. Systems theory can be used to support, evaluate, change, and guide nursing practice. As the largest of the groups of professional provides in the health care delivery system, nurses can and should have a tremendous impact on the quality of care within that system. As nurses, we can utilize the resources of technology and the knowledge explosion to the benefit of our clients, if we are willing.

References

1. Bertalanffy, L.v. (1968). General Systems Theory. New York: Braziller.
2. Bertalanffy, L.v. (1975). Perspectives on General Systems Theory. New York: Braziller, p. 153.
3. Boulding, K.E. (1968). General systems theory: The skeleton of science. In: W. Buckley, ed., Modern Systems Research for the Behavioral Sciences. Chicago: Aldine.

4. Baker, F. (1970). General systems theory, research, and medical care. In: A. Sheldon, F. Baker, and C.P. McLaughlin, eds., Systems and Medical Care. Cambridge, MA: M.I.T. Press.

5. LaPatra, J.W. (1975). Health Care Delivery Systems. Springfield, IL: Charles C Thomas.

6. Miller, J.G. (1978). Living Systems. New York: McGraw-Hill, p. 25.

7. Hazzard, M.E. (1971). An overview of systems theory. Nursing Clinics of North America 6(3):385-393.

8. Wang, R.M. and Hawkins, J.W. (1980). Interpersonal feedback for nurse supervisors. Supervisor Nurse 11(1):26-28.

9. Miller, G.A. (1970). General systems approach to the patient and his environment. In: A Sheldon, F. Baker, and C.P. McLaughlin, eds, Systems and Medical Care. Cambridge, MA: The M.I.T. Press, p. 83.

10. King, I.M. (1976). The health care system: Nursing intervention system. In: H.H. Werley, A. Zuzich, M. Zajkowksi, and A.D. Zagornik, eds., Health Research: The Systems Approach. New York: Springer, pp. 51-60.

11. Passos, J.Y. (1976). Systems approach and evaluation of quality of care in an urban hospital. In: H.H. Werley, A. Zuzich, M. Zajkowksi, and A.D. Zagornik, eds., Health Research: The Systems Approach. New York: Springer, pp. 193-200.

12. Putt, A.M. (1978). General Systems Theory Applied to Nursing. Boston: Little Brown, pp. 31-35.

13. Headline news. (1992). American Journal of Nursing 92(7):9.

2

The Organization of Health Care Delivery in the United States

An Historical Perspective

Health care in colonial America was the responsibility of those who were chosen because of "skill and fitness to care for the sick," according to early records. At the Plymouth colony, Samuel Fuller, one of the deacons, acted as physician, and his wife was the first midwife. Clergymen were often also physicians in the New England settlements (1, p.100). Accounts of early seventeenth-century colonial America list 2 women and 74 men as physicians (in some historical accounts, the women are referred to as midwives) (2, p. 5). This new nation, with its multitude of problems due to disease, weather, and the grueling daily pace necessary for survival, depended on women to provide health care in the same manner as they had in their homelands. They served as healers, lay midwives, and untrained nurses.

The Dutch East India Company established a cottage hospital for its company in 1658. Eventually, it became Bellevue Hospital (3, p. 140). In 1731, Blockley Hospital, later Philadelphia General, was established. Thereafter, over the remainder of the eighteenth century, numerous well-known hospitals were founded in the larger towns: Charity Hospital in New Orleans (1737);

Pennsylvania Hospital in Philadelphia (1751); Eastern State Hospital in Williamsburg, Virginia (1770); New York Hospital (1771); the Philadelphia Dispensary (1786); and the Boston Dispensary (1796) (1, pp. 110-111).

Paralleling the development of hospitals was the establishment of schools of medicine. In 1713, Boston, then the largest city in the colonies, had only one university-trained physician for its 100,000 residents. Although it was already a well-established practice in Europe for one to possess a university degree in order to call oneself a doctor, anyone with any medical training, or none at all, could do so in the colonies (4, pp. 6-8).

The first medical schools were established in Philadelphia (1765) and New York (1767).[1] Since demand exceeded supply, however, the apprentice system continued and flourished. Proprietary medical schools sprang up to attempt to meet the demand. By 1876, 64 medical colleges existed out of 80 established to that year in the U.S. Many of these were proprietary and the quality declined.

After the establishment of the first Nightingale schools of nursing in the United States in 1873, hospitals jumped on the bandwagon. They saw these schools as an answer to problems of staffing and providing patient care. By 1880, there were 15 nurse training schools; by 1890, 35; and by 1900, 432 hospital schools produced 3,456 graduate nurses (5).

Evolution of the Role of Local Governments in Health Care

It seems appropriate at this point to diverge from a general discussion of the history of health care providers and facilities to focus on the evolution of government's role in health care delivery since the two are parallel. Local, federal, and state involvement will be discussed in that order, as they evolved historically.

---

[1] Kings College Medical School, founded on November 2, 1767, is now the College of Physicians and Surgeons. The Medical School of the College of Philadelphia, founded on November 14, 1765, is now the University of Pennsylvania.

From an historical perspective, health care and medical care were first perceived as local problems. Almshouses and poorhouses were established early in the eighteenth century under local aegis. The Publick House and House of Corrections, established in New York City in 1735, is a typical example. That it incarcerated both criminals and the poor was no accident, for the latter were, through their poverty, also offenders of society. The Philadelphia General Hospital was, at first, an almshouse. Bellevue Hospital was a pesthouse in early years, designed to protect society from victims of the plague. Lunatic asylums, too, were founded, not to help the mentally ill but to protect the public (6, pp. 43, 45-46).

Epidemics in the eighteenth and nineteenth centuries forced local authorities to undertake active measures to protect the public. Between 1832 and 1840, 4,500 persons in New York City succumbed to cholera. Vigorous protective measures, including health examinations and quarantine of immigrants, reduced the number to nine by 1883. Thus, local health efforts led to the development of local health departments, often established in response to epidemics in an effort to protect the public. Today, in every state some responsibility for health is delegated to local authorities.

Miller and his co-workers reported in 1977 that, through a survey of public health statutes of all 50 states, they identified some 44 specific services or functions that were assigned to local health departments. These ranged from controlling communicable disease and collecting vital statistics, to enforcing environmental and food regulations, designing specific programs for a variety of conditions, and providing direct services such as home care, family planning and public health nursing care (7). Since 1977, these basic functions have not changed, but have expanded in response to such social problems as AIDS, homelessness, urban violence, family violence, and substance abuse (61). To these have been added health promotion in response to the health objectives for the year 2000 (62, 63).

Some local communities or counties operate public hospitals through their local public health structure. These public hospitals are increasingly experiencing financial difficulties due to their clients' inability to pay for services. In 1990, 1,444 rural community and urban hospitals in the country were owned by state or local governments (51). Closing these hospitals or cutting back in their services can have a profound effect on health care delivery since these institutions handle a great number of outpatient and emergency visits and act as the family doctor for countless citizens.

Organizational structures vary in different regions of the country. Some states require that local governments establish and conduct a local health department and others permit them to do so (61). Some states have programs for model standards for local health departments (65). The majority of local health departments exercise jurisdiction over a single unit of local government, be it a city, town, or county. The predominant local unit in New England and the middle Atlantic states is the town, whereas county, multi-county, or city/county jurisdictions are more common in the mountain, South Atlantic, and East South Central regions (9, pp. 931-933).

A trend toward merging small local health departments is increasing in impetus due to economic constraints. A population base of several small towns or counties can more easily support professionals for full-time service, justify applications for grants and other outside funds, and avoid duplication of services. There is also a trend toward a broader role for local government in providing direct care services (18b). When local governments cannot or will not maintain local health departments, the state can manage or control districts, serving as a local presence (61).

Funds for local departments come from federal, state, and local budgets (11, 18a). The largest proportion comes from local sources followed by state and federal sources; the remainder is generated by fees for services. It is difficult to pinpoint sources of monies which may come via agencies such as welfare departments and which may originate as federal funds (9, p. 933).

Services provided by local health departments vary widely. They may include any or all of the following: immunization programs, environmental surveillance, tuberculosis and other communicable disease control, maternal child health, school health, sexually transmitted disease control, home care, chronic disease programs, family planning, traffic safety prevention and health promotion programs, food protection, nutritional services, vehicular and non-vehicular injury control, and ambulatory care (9, p. 934; 62; 63; 64; 65).

In some instances, the local health authorities may be the sole provider of one or more services within the areas of jurisdiction. Some interesting findings concerning priorities emerged in Miller's study. Health code enforcement ranked high in New England and the Middle Atlantic states, whereas direct delivery of medical services ranked highest in the South Atlantic states and lowest in New England and the Middle Atlantic states (9, p. 934).

Staffing varies widely. Many local health officers are physicians; the rest have degrees in public health or have a BS, BA, MA, or MS degree (18c). Nurses may be employed by local health departments for a variety of roles. Small health departments sometimes choose to contract with local visiting nurse associations (these are voluntary, nonprofit, private organizations) for nursing services rather than hire nurses for public health functions. At the local level, nurses may participate in a wide range of activities including screening; disease prevention and health promotion programs; home care; communicable disease case finding and follow-up; poison control center follow-up; inspection and licensure of facilities; health education; and programs having to do with maternal and child care, AIDS, mental illness, occupational hazards, family planning, school health, care of the indigent and homeless, immunizations, housing inspection, and emergency and ambulance services.

The first visiting nursing association was established in Boston, which was also the first city to begin a community nursing service. Baltimore and New York both hired nurses for tuberculosis work in 1903. By 1906, 34 nurses in nine cities were employed in tuberculosis prevention. New York was the first city in 1902, to hire school nurses (3, pp. 320-327).

Evolution of the Role of the Federal Government in Health Care

The Constitution does not define a role for the federal government in

Table 2.1   Legislative Branch — Health Affairs

Structure	Function(s)
Congressional Budget Office	Provides Congress with detailed budget information and studies budget impact of alternative policies.
Congressional Research Service	Department of Library of Congress. Provides resources for its members.
General Accounting Office	Directly responsible to Congress. Conducts independent reviews, audits, and investigations of federal agencies.
Office of Technology Assessment	Advisory to Congress. Provides objective information on ramifications of policy choices affecting the use of technology; health is one area; other areas related to health are the ocean, transportation, energy, food.

health care either as a provider of services or as a payer for services rendered by others. The official entry of the federal government into the health care arena was in 1798. In that year, an act of Congress established the Marine Hospital Service for the Relief of Sick and Disabled Seamen. This service was financed by a monthly tax of 20 cents against each seaman's wages. Similar hospitals were established in Virginia in 1801 and in Boston in 1803; until 1884 these continued to be financed by the seamen. After that time, a tax was levied on merchant marine tonnage to support the hospitals, and in 1905 the federal government began to support these services out of general tax revenues (6, p. 44).

The role of the federal government in health care has increased dramatically since those early years nearly two centuries ago. Today, the role of the federal government involves all three branches. Congress, the legislative branch, has been very active, particularly in recent years, in considering and enacting health care legislation.

The executive branch administers federal programs for health care, beginning with certain programs originating directly from the

Office of the President and those under the aegis of the various cabinet-level departments. The judiciary branch adjudicates in cases related to health care and human rights (11, p. 337). Perhaps one of the most publicized judicial decisions affecting health care in recent years was the 1973 Supreme Court ruling on abortion, known as Roe v. Wade.

The general functions of the federal government in health care may be summarized as follows: providing direct care for certain groups such as Native Americans, the military and their dependents, and veterans; safeguarding the public's health by regulating quarantine and immigration and the marketing of food, drugs, and biologicals; preventing environmental hazards; giving grants in aid to states, local areas, and individuals; and conducting and supporting research.

Federal involvement in health care may be said to begin with the Office of the President, to whom the Office of Management and the Budget reports directly. All federal funds to support health-related activities are generated in the Office of Management and the Budget. A number of programs in independent agencies report, or have reported during their tenure, directly to the President. Examples include the now defunct Office of Economic Opportunity founded in 1964 and the Drug Abuse Prevention Program launched in 1971. Cabinet-level departments function under the Office of the President in the executive branch of government. Most are in one way or another involved in administering health-related programs.

Selected examples of the health-related functions of the various cabinet-level departments and their component parts are listed below. Some of these departments exist as political whims and fancies and in the future may be subsumed under other departments in efforts to curb costs.

Department of Agriculture

This department administers a number of programs that are related to the health of our nation's citizens. Among these are the school breakfast programs, nonfood assistance for school food service programs, the national school lunch and milk programs, and the child care and summer food programs (10, 12). The food stamp program, begun in 1961, is under its direction. So is WIC, the Special Supplemental Food Program for Women, Infants, and Children. This program provides for nutritious food supplements for pregnant, postpartum, and lactating women and for children up to age five who are certified as nutritionally at risk. It also allows WIC participants to use benefits to purchase fresh produce at farmers' markets (10, 13). Various other food programs under the department provide food for schools, summer food programs, the Commodity Supplemental Food distribution, charitable institutions, camps, the elderly, disaster victims, needy families, homeless persons, and for families on some Indian reservations. The Nutrition Education and Training Program provides education on nutrition for children and inservice education for teachers and food service personnel (10, 12).

Programs such as these are funded at the discretion of the administration and Congress. Their existence is threatened in times of budget cutting and revamping of social programs.

In addition to food programs, the Department of Agriculture's Food Safety and Quality Service is responsible for inspecting meat, eggs, and poultry, and for monitoring supplies of farm products and regulating labeling of meat products (14). The Federal Grain Inspection and Animal and Plant Inspection Services help to assure a safe food supply. Forest and Soil Conservation Services are important to the environment.

Department of Defense

The Department of Defense assumes responsibility for the health care of active-duty military personnel and their dependents at home and abroad and of survivors and retirees and their dependents and their eligible dependents and survivors. Civilians in need of emergency care who are in close proximity to a military health care facility can also be beneficiaries (66). It is incumbent upon this department's military health care delivery system to provide health services for all active-duty personnel regardless of where they may be located. For dependents, survivors, and retirees, however, these services are rendered according to priority and availability of services.

There has been a move in recent years to regionalize and coordinate health services among the three military branches to avoid duplication and to maximize economy. With the end of the Cold War, there is also discussion of consolidating the military forces instead of continuing to support three active branches. In addition to client care, the military health services are responsible for environmental sanitation, including safe water and food supplies, in areas where military forces are stationed both in peacetime and during mobilization and war (66). (See Chapter 4 for a more detailed description of the military subsystem of health care.)

Department of Housing and Urban Development (HUD)

Concerned with urban development in low income areas, this department has helped to fund neighborhood health centers through a bill passed in 1966 allowing long-term loans for financing facilities. The monies have been used to build, rehabilitate, equip, and furnish structures for the group practice of medicine, dentistry, or optometry. This has included nonprofit groups or organizations establishing neighborhood health facilities. HUD also sponsors a program of mortgage insurance to attract major private capital for building and rehabilitating hospitals and other health care facilities. Eligibility is determined through the Department of Health and Human Services, using Hill-Burton standards. (The Hill-Burton Act is discussed in Chapter 3.) A similar program is available for constructing new nursing homes and rehabilitating existing structures, including those for intermediate and day care.

Newer programs include congregate housing, supportive housing for persons with disabilities, emergency shelters for the homeless, transitional housing, and housing for seniors and persons with AIDS (8).

Department of the Interior

Assuming responsibility as guardian of our natural resources, the work of the Department of the Interior is important in maintaining or restoring an optimal geographic health environment in our nation to assure preservation of our land and water resources, fish and wildlife, and recreation areas (20). The Bureau of Mines and the Bureau of Indian Affairs are part of the Department of the Interior.

The Bureau of Mines, under this department, is responsible for controlling health and safety hazards in mining. The department is also responsible for Native American education, national environmental studies, and for water resources research (19).

Federal involvement in the health care of miners dates to a 1946 agreement signed by the then Secretary of the Interior and the United Mine Workers president, John L. Lewis, which created a United Mine Workers' Welfare and Retirement Fund to be supported by coal royalty payments. The fund was subsequently used to build hospitals and to operate them as well as clinics. By the 1960s the number of coal miners had decreased sharply and Appalachian Regional Hospitals, Inc., a new group supported by grant and loan funds, took over the miners' regional hospital chain. Because of rising costs and fewer miners, in 1977 deductibles became necessary. Thus, miners' benefits have become more limited and the struggle for health services has become an unresolved issue. In 1977, the Mining Enforcement and Safety Administration was transferred to the Department of Labor and was, as of March 1978, designated the Mine Safety and Health Administration.

When the Interior Department was first established in 1849, the *Bureau of Indian Affairs* was transferred to it from the War Department (19, p.3\0. There it remains, but in 1955 health services for Native Americans were transferred to the Public Health Service.

Department of Labor

This department was created in 1913 to promote and protect the welfare of employees. It is responsible for enforcing laws which protect the health and safety of the nation's workers, as well as their jobs and pension rights (15). It sets standards for child labor to protect the health and welfare of children. The department also assumes responsibility for such things as standards for migrant housing and enforcement of the Fair Labor Standards Act (1938) as amended in 1977 (18). It also includes:

The Mine Safety and Health Administration (MSHA) falls under this department. This agency issues and enforces the standards of the Mine Safety and Health Act of 1977. Its Health and Safety Analysis Center in Denver collects and analyzes data from mine accidents. MSHA also trains miners, administrators, and instructors for health and safety courses (18).

The Bureau of Labor Statistics of the Labor Department keeps data on job safety and health.

The Labor Department's *Employment Standards Administration* administers compensation programs for federal employees and certain workers (including coal miners suffering from black lung), maritime workers, and certain other groups who are eligible for benefits due to job related injuries, diseases, and death (16).

The Occupational Safety and Health Administration (OSHA) of the Department of Labor was established by an act of Congress in 1970. It is designed to encourage employees and employers to reduce hazards and institute health and safety programs, establish a record-keeping system to monitor accidents and illness, develop and enforce mandatory standards for health and safety, and push states to assume responsibility for programs (17). OSHA cooperates with the Food and Drug Administration, the Environmental Protection Agency, the Food Safety and Quality Service of the Agriculture Department, and the Consumer Products Safety Commission. The 1970 act also mandated creation of the National Institute of Occupational Safety and Health (NIOSH) to research hazards related to industry and to prepare health standards and recommend them to OSHA (18). In 1986, an evaluation project was initiated by NIOSH to examine its surveillance activities (67).

Department of Justice

The Department of Justice offers law enforcement assistance for control of narcotic and dangerous drug traffic, and assists in educating the public on drug abuse (21).

The *Federal Bureau of Prisons (BOP)* is an agency of this department. The Public Health Service provides health care professionals, including nurses, to provide health care for the more than 47,000 inmates in 57 institutions. It employs 450 nurse practitioners and 250 other nurses (32).

The *Immigration and Naturalization Service (INS)* is also part of Justice and provides health care to detainees. Nurses and nurse practitioners are part of the health care team in its eight medical facilities (32).

Department of State

The Department of State helps facilitate educational exchanges and assists students from foreign countries to enroll in studies in the health professions (12, p. 470). Health care professionals work in the Office of Medical Services to care for State Department employees and their families abroad (29).

Department of Commerce

Certain monitoring and control programs for marine and atmospheric pollution fall under the aegis of this department. It also provides grants and loans for the construction of water and waste treatment facilities and for sewer and water lines.

Its major agency is the *National Oceanic and Atmospheric Administration (NOAA)*. The Public Health Service provides care for the Health Services Program of NOAA for its commissioned corps and their dependents (32).

The *Bureau of the Census* also falls under this department. The census is very important for planning services such as child care and senior centers at the local level. Census data also help in planning health programs by identifying groups that might need services such as seniors and children, as well as new immigrants (22).

Department of Energy

The Department of Energy was established in 1977 and is involved in promoting health and preventing illness through research on waste management, overseeing reactor and nonreactor nuclear facilities, implementing energy conservation measures by hospitals, and managing programs for radioactive waste management (23). The department also assures environmental health by monitoring the safety of new energy technologies.

Department of Transportation

This department is concerned with transportation safety and the impact of modes of transport on environment. This includes marine environment protection and boat safety, pollution control, safety related to aviation, problems of noise pollution and vibration, safety related to motor vehicles, and railway safety. The *Transportation Systems Center* is charged with planning for the future of transportation through research and coordination of government efforts at the federal, state, and local levels, academia, and private industry (24).

Department of the Treasury

Two components of this department have functions related to the health of our citizens. They are:

The *Bureau of Alcohol, Tobacco, and Firearms* which regulates these three industries and investigates violations of federal laws (25).

The Customs Service which is involved in narcotics traffic control and has certain shoreline and marine protection functions. It also enforces laws regarding animal, plant, and bird quarantines.

Department of Education

This cabinet-level department of our federal government, established in 1980, is responsible for programs for the educationally deprived: migrant farm workers, the handicapped, the neglected, and the delinquent. It provides for alcohol and drug abuse education, for environmental education, and for vocational education for the handicapped, including the blind, and the rehabilitation of disabled adults. Special training projects include biomedical services and consumer education. The department offers basic educational opportunity grants which may help students gain first-level or preprofessional education for health professions (26).

Department of Veterans Affairs

In 1989, the *Veterans Administration* became the newest cabinet-level department. It oversees 172 VA medical centers, 233 outpatient clinics, and dozens of other facilities. There are 58 regional offices for veterans affairs and 112 national cemeteries under its jurisdiction. As an employer of over 240,000 persons, it is second in size to the Department of Defense. Its three major program areas are medical care, benefits, and cemeteries. In Chapter 4, nursing in the VA system is described in more detail (68).

Department of Health and Human Services (HHS)

When the new Department of Education was born on May 4, 1980, the Department of Health and Human Services (HHS) was created out of the 27-year-old Department of Health, Education, and Welfare which, in turn, had been a child of the Federal Security Agency born in 1953. The component parts of HHS are the Health Care Financing Administration, the Social Security Administration, the Office of Human Development Services, the Public Health Service, the Office of Community Services, and the Office of Child Support Enforcement.

The Health Care Financing Administration, organized in 1977, is charged with overseeing Medicare and Medicaid. In 1981, Carolyne Davis became the first nurse to head this agency.

The Social Security Administration collects data on costs and expenditures for health and is responsible for Social Security retirement benefits, certain federal welfare programs, unemployment insurance, old age insurance, survivors and disability insurance, supplemental security income for the aged, and benefits for the blind and disabled.

The Office of Human Development Services is responsible for programs for young people, Native Americans, Alaskan Natives, families in need, child development programs, and Head Start. In 1912, the Children's Bureau was founded by an act of Congress under the initiative of Lillian D. Wald (3, p. 33); this bureau is now subsumed under HHS's Office of Human Development Services.

The Public Health Service. This is the oldest of Health and Human Service's component agencies. It was created in 1798 as the Marine Hospital for the Relief of Sick and Disabled Seamen. All quarantine became the responsibility of the Marine Hospital Service in 1893 (6, pp. 44-45). In 1912, this service was renamed the Public Health Service.

In 1854, Congress allocated 10 million acres in each state, the income from which was to be used to support asylums for the insane, and also 2.5 million acres per state to support deaf mutes and the blind (6, p. 45). By the end of the Civil War, the government had taken over Freedman's Hospital to care for ex-slaves and St. Elizabeth's as an asylum for the mentally ill, both in the District of Columbia. A National Board of Health was organized in 1878 to help control epidemics, but died for lack of funds in 1883. In 1887, a laboratory was opened on Staten Island in New York to do bacteriological research; it eventually moved to the District of Columbia to become the National Institutes of Health.

Under the reorganization scheme of the Califano administration implemented in 1978, the principal officer of the Public Health Service is the Surgeon General, who is an Assistant Secretary of Health. (See Figure 2.1). In 1982, Faye G. Abdellah became the Deputy Surgeon General, the first woman and first nurse in that position. When she retired, Dr. O. Marie Henry became Deputy Surgeon General, and when Dr. Antonia Novello was appointed Surgeon General and Dr. Bernadine Healy became the director of NIH, for the first time in history all three positions were filled by women.

The Agencies Within the Public Health Service

The Substance Abuse and Mental Health Services Administration oversees three component centers: the Center for Substance Abuse Treatment, the Center for Substance Abuse Prevention, and the Center for Mental Health Services. Under Public Law 101-321 (the ADAMHA Reorganization Act of 1992), the Alcohol, Drug Abuse, and Mental Health Administration (ADAMHA) of the Public Health Service became this new agency. The three research institutes formerly under ADAMHA were transferred as separate institutes into the National Institutes of Health. The Center for Mental Health Services (CMHS) coordinates the federal role in prevention and treatment of mental illness and promotion of mental health and administers grants, programs, and clinical training for health care professionals and paraprofessionals. Mental Health Services block grants are administered by CMHS and those for substance abuse services are administered under the Center for Substance Abuse Treatment (CSAT). All programs for substance abuse prevention are administered under the Center for Substance Abuse Prevention (CSAP) (71).

The National Institute of Mental Health conducts research, explores special areas, investigates psychopharmacology, and   is engaged in the education of care providers. It also administers St. Elizabeth's, the federal psychiatric hospital in Washington, D.C.

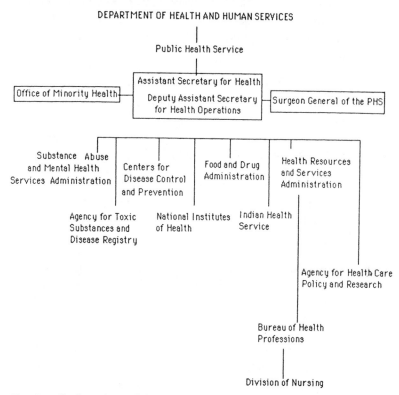

Fig. 2.1. Outline chart of the Public Health Service, Department of Health and Human Services.

The Centers for Disease Control and Prevention (CDC), headquartered in Atlanta, Georgia, is the child of the Communicable Disease Center, founded in 1946, and grandchild of an agency called Malaria Control in War Areas that was founded during World War II to coordinate the control of malaria and other diseases. The CDC is responsible for following disease trends, for coordinating its activities with those of other countries, and for providing leadership to state and local areas for communicable disease control. It provides laboratory services for unusual problems; supplies rare vaccines and drugs not otherwise available; participates in training occupational safety and health professionals; responds to calls for help from states when epidemics occur; provides smoking health education; is involved in health promotion programs, parenting education, STD and AIDS education; and is concerned with rat control and lead screening programs. In 1992, "Prevention" was added to its name to reflect the evolution of its mission in the control and prevention of disease, injury, and disability (30).

The Centers for Disease Control and Prevention also works on noncommunicable diseases and occupational health concerns. Its Epidemic Intelligence Service employs health care professionals who might be assigned to work from the offices of a local or state health department as well as at the CDC. There are several important programs within CDC. *The Center for Environmental Health and Injury Control* is concerned with preventing illness and premature death from hazards outside the work place. Professionals assigned to the *Center for Health Promotion and Education* are engaged in epidemiologic studies on health risks of behavior choices in order to develop intervention programs. The *Center for Infectious Diseases* focuses on research and control of endemic and epidemic infectious diseases. Health care professionals in the *Center for Prevention Services* work on one of the several focus areas: tuberculosis, immunizations, sexually transmitted diseases, refuge health and foreign quarantine, diabetes and related chronic diseases, dental disease, quarantine, and health services analysis. The *National Institute for Occupational Safety and Health,* known as NIOSH, is concerned with the safety and health of American workers and makes recommendations to OSHA and the Mine Safety and Health Administration, both part of the Department of Labor. CDC also trains health professionals through the Training and Laboratory Program Office. (29).

In 1946, the National Office of Vital Statistics of the Bureau of the Census was transferred to the U.S. Public Health Service and was merged in 1960 with the National Health Survey, founded in 1956, to form the *National Center for Health Statistics*, part of the CDC. At the

National Center for Health Statistics, researchers design and implement national health surveys, collect and analyze the nation's health and vital statistics, disseminate information, and provide technical assistance here and abroad (49).

The Food and Drug Administration (FDA) is charged with enforcement of legislation to protect the public from unsafe consumer goods, foods, medicines, vaccines and other biologicals, and from radiation from X-ray machines. Most of its activities have evolved from five major acts: the Federal Food, Drug, and Cosmetic Act; the Fair Packaging and Labeling Act; the Radiation Control for Health and Safety Act; the Public Health Service Act; and the Medical Devices Amendments. The FDA's component bureaus oversee the safety of foods, biologicals, blood and blood products, drugs, medical devices, diagnostic products, veterinary medicine (including drugs adminis-tered to animals), devices emitting radiation, and the safety of electronic products including TV sets, microwave ovens, lasers, and ultraviolet lights. They also oversee research in toxicology.

There are those who believe that the FDA is often too cautious and thereby holds up approval of certain medications long after they are in common use in other countries. Others disagree and cite instances when harm was averted because the agency moved slowly. An example of this is the caution that was exercised in approving thalidomide before its effects were known. Thus, few babies born in the country were affected by the malformations the drugs causes. In 1985, an Action Plan for FDA was initiated to address problems caused by a dramatic increase in the work of the FDA (31).

The Health Resources and Services Administration (HRSA) has as its responsibility the identification, development, and optimal utilization of the nation's health resources. To this end, HRSA collaborates with health providers and with educational and service facilities. It funds AIDS care demonstration centers and administers the National Organ Transplant Act. It concentrates on providing an adequate supply of health care providers and minimizing maldistribu-tion of professionals. Its *Bureau of Maternal and Child Health and*

Resources Development awards funds to the states for maternal/child health promotion. Its *Bureau of Health Care Delivery and Assistance* is one of the components of the federal government most directly involved in service provision by directing personnel and resources to underserved areas. It conducts research, provides some educational programs for students in health professions, and is involved in programs to improve emergency medical services and monitor rural health issues across the country. It administers the National Health Service Corps, including its scholarship and loan repayment programs. Since the Corps was founded in 1972, l6,000 health care professionals have served in underserved areas (69).

HRSA's *Bureau of Health Professions* (previously called the Bureau of Health Manpower) monitors training, supply distribution, and conduct of health professionals. It includes offices for program development, program support, debt management, and data analysis and management. Divisions include Associated and Dental Health Professions, Medicine, Nursing, Student Assistance, and Disadvantaged Assistance.

The *Division of Nursing,* which falls under HRSA's Bureau of Health Professions, was established in 1919 and was first headed by

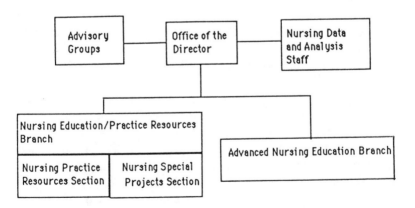

Fig. 2.2. Division of Nursing, 1992.

Lucy Minnigerode (3, p. 347). A graduate of Bellevue, she had served abroad, then as a Red Cross staff member, and then as an inspector of Marine hospitals under the Public Health Service. In 1919, she was appointed superintendent of nurses of the PHS (33).

The Division of Nursing attempts to increase the availability and quality of health services by expanding the role of nursing in health care. It administers the Nurse Training Act of 1971 (reauthorized annually by Congress through the budget process), which is designated to provide advanced training for nurses for expanded roles in primary care (nurse practitioners) and teaching, and to accelerate recruitment of minorities into nursing. It provides aid for students and schools of nursing and enables graduate nursing students to qualify for nurse traineeships. In 1985, research activities were moved to NIH with the authorization of the National Center for Nursing Research (NCNR). In recent years, division funds have been cut, but nurse training funds were available as of the 1993/1994 budget. The Division of Nursing also reviews nursing issues, prepares publications about its studies, and is a clearing house for information on nursing (34).

The Indian Health Service became the seventh agency in the Public Health Service in 1988. It provides comprehensive health services, including primary, emergency and preventive care, to over one million Native Americans and Alaska Natives in 500 tribal groups. It assists tribes to develop their health programs and serves as a principal federal advocate for Native Americans in the health field. A more complete discussion of the IHS is in chapter 4 (29, 32).

The National Institutes of Health (NIH) is a medical research center comprised of 16 research institutes, the National Library of Medicine, the National Center for Biomedical Communication, and a 540-bed hospital. The institutes are as follows: Aging; Alcohol Abuse and Alcoholism; Allergy and Infectious Disease; Arthritis; Cancer; Child Health and Human Development; Dental Research; Diabetes, Digestive and Kidney Diseases; Drug Abuse; Environmental Health Sciences; Eye; General Medical Studies; Heart, Lung, and Blood;

Mental Health; the National Institute for Nursing Research (created out of the National Center for Nursing Research in June, 1993), and Neurological and Communicative Disorders and Stroke. All except Environmental Health Sciences (at Research Triangle Park, North Carolina) are located in Bethesda, Maryland.

The nearly 14,000 persons employed by NIH are engaged in some 2,500 research projects. Its National Library of Medicine lists *Index Medicus* among its publications (29, 32). The Fogarty International Center, also part of NIH, coordinates efforts in biomedical research and houses foreign scholars. The Clinical Center of NIH employs many nurses as members of the research and client care teams. Nurses may either be appointed to NIH as commissioned officers in the Public Health Service or they may be civilians with civil service status under the Federal Civil Service (35).

The years between 1945 and 1965 were boom years for research. Many benefits were derived from the enormous amount of money poured into research by the federal government. Not only were research programs expanded and space increased, but thousands of researchers were trained. There were also some long-term detrimental effects, e.g.: the rapid expansion was not based on any clear mission or philosophy; grants that were made for particular disease research often depended on the personal experience of leading politicians; and more research was done on cures for cancer than on its causes (36).

In 1990, the General Accounting Office (GAO) issued a scathing report on the exclusion of women from medical research projects. As a result, the Women's Health Equity Act was introduced into the 101st Congress and passed by the 102nd. The Office of Research on Women's Health was created at NIH as a result of this legislation. Concurrently, the first woman director of NIH was appointed (28).

The Agency for Toxic Substances and Disease Registry is another agency of the Public Health Service. It is responsible for investigating the possible toxic effects of over 60,000 chemicals. It also works to develop more advanced testing methods, coordinates research and testing efforts of all the PHS agencies, and communicates its findings to the government, industry, labor, environmental groups, and the public and public interest groups (32).

Table 2.2   Public Health Service Regional Offices

Region	States	Address
I	Connecticut, Maine, Massachusetts, New Hampshire, Rhode Island Vermont	John F. Kennedy Federal Bldg. Boston, MA 02203
II	New Jersey, New York, Puerto Rico, Virgin Islands	Jacob K. Javits Federal Bldg. 26 Federal Plaza New York, NY 10278
III	Delaware, District of Columbia, Maryland, Pennsylvania, Virginia, West Virginia	3535 Market St. P.O. Box 13716 Philadelphia, PA 19101
IV	Alabama, Florida, Georgia, Kentucky, Mississippi, North Carolina, South Carolina, Tennessee	101 Marietta Tower Atlanta, GA 30323
V	Illinois, Indiana, Michigan, Minnesota, Ohio, Wisconsin	105 West Adams St. Chicago, IL 60603
VI	Arkansas, Louisiana, New Mexico, Oklahoma, Texas	1200 Main Tower Bldg. Dallas, TX 75202
VII	Iowa, Kansas, Missouri, Nebraska	601 East 12th St. Kansas City, MO 64106
VIII	Colorado, Montana, North Dakota, South Dakota, Utah, Wyoming	1961 Stout St. Denver, CO 80294-3538
IX	American Samoa, Arizona, California, Guam, Hawaii, Nevada, Trust Territory of the Pacific Islands	50 United Nations Plaza San Francisco, CA 94102
X	Alaska, Idaho, Oregon, Washington	Blanchard Plaza Bldg. 2201 Sixth Ave. Seattle, WA 98121

The Agency for Health Care Policy and Research (AHCPR) was established in 1989 as part of the Public Health Service, superseding the National Center for Health Services Research and Health Care Technology Assessment. It is the responsibility of this new agency to enhance the effectiveness, quality and appropriateness of health care services and access to services through research and promotion of improvements in clinical practice, and in the organization, financing, and delivery of health care services (70).

The Public Health Service also has 10 regional offices responsible for implementing Public Health Service policies and programs, overseeing grants and contracts, and providing technical assistance to state and local health officers (see Table 2.2).

Independent Agencies

A number of independent federal agencies are also concerned and involved with the health of the nation.

ACTION, created in 1971, is the umbrella agency for such volunteer programs as VISTA, the Peace Corps, the Senior Companion Program, the Retired Senior Volunteer Program, the Foster Grandparent Program, ACTION Drug Alliance, and Student Community Service Program. VISTA workers have been involved in health and environmental improvement projects, as have Peace Corps volunteers. The other programs have included or do include health and nutrition among their targets (27).

The Appalachian Regional Commission (ARC) is an agency concerned with the 13-state Appalachian area. Among its activities are the administration of health and child development programs for the target group, and the funding of environmental projects (sewers, water, solid waste).

The Community Services Administration, which replaced the Office of Economic Opportunity, is responsible for certain community action programs, some of which deal with medical care, nutrition, and housing.

The Consumer Product Safety Commission, established in 1972, is concerned with the safety of consumer products and with preventing accidents associated with their use.

The Environmental Protection Agency (EPA), established in 1970, is charged with controlling and enforcing antipollution laws and, as a foundation, conducts research on control standards and the effects of pollution on humans. It is concerned with air and water quality, solid waste disposal control, pesticide regulation, radiation hazard control, and toxic substances.

The Federal Maritime Commission regulates waterborne commerce and assures that vessel owners assume fiscal accountability for water pollution due to oil spills, and so forth.

The Federal Mine Safety and Health Review Commission is the adjudicating body when enforcement actions of the Secretary of Labor are contested.

The Federal Trade Commission (FTC) prevents false or deceptive advertising, regulates packaging and labeling of selected products including foods, drugs, and cosmetics, and regulates cigarette advertising.

The General Services Administration operates the Consumer Information Center and publishes a catalog of federal publications on many topics including health.

National Aeronautics and Space Administration (NASA) conducts life science research. Physicians and other health care professionals work at NASA, mostly in occupational health (11).

The National Science Foundation supports all manner of research including that concerned with health, safety, and the environment.

The National Transportation Safety Board conducts investigations when accidents occur, be they marine, rail, air, highway, or pipeline.

The Nuclear Regulatory Commission, established in 1974, handles all licensing and regulatory functions formerly handled by the Atomic Energy Commission.

The Occupational Safety and Health Review Commission adjudicates enforcement actions of OSHA.

The Small Business Administration has functions which protect consumers and provide for occupational health and safety.

The Tennessee Valley Authority, in existence since 1933, is concerned with environmental protection and planning, and conducts health programs.

Quasi-Official Agencies

Several quasi-official agencies that are concerned with health are:

The National Academy of Sciences, established by an act of Congress in 1863, serves in an advisory capacity to the federal government and is engaged in research related to child development, substance abuse, environmental impact on health, and other health-related topics.

The Smithsonian Institution, which is an independent trust, sponsors research on such topics as human nutrition, preservation of the environment, and disease prevention.

The American National Red Cross, established by an act of Congress in 1882, owes its existence in this country to the efforts of Clara Barton (37). Jane Delano, a graduate of Bellevue Hospital School of Nursing and at one time a recruiter of nurses for the Red Cross, became chairperson of the National Committee on Red Cross Nursing Service in 1909, the year of its founding. She co-authored the first text on home care of the sick and served as an active leader in Red Cross nursing until her death in 1919 (38).

Today, nurses serve the Red Cross in both voluntary and paid staff positions. They are engaged in activities ranging from disaster health services to screening programs, blood bank work, instructing nurses' aides and the public in a wide variety of subjects, and administering programs (38). Nurses symbolize the Red Cross to many persons both here and abroad.

Evolution of the Role of the States in Health Care

States became involved in and concerned about the health of their citizens as a result of the epidemics of the nineteenth century. In response to the yellow fever epidemic of 1853, the Louisiana legislature established, in 1855, the first permanent state board of health in the United States and set up a quarantine system (41). In 1869, Massachusetts became the first state to define its legal responsibilities for health. Although impetus was provided by the Shattuck Report on Health in Boston in 1850, it nonetheless took 19 years for the implementation of its recommendation that a board of health be established. The report, by Lemuel Shattuck, a bookseller and publisher, became the foundation for recording health statistics in the United States (42).

Since, under the Constitution, states are delegated police power to enact and enforce laws to protect their citizens, they have legal authority in matters of health (11, p. 335). "The state has the power to enact and enforce laws to protect and promote health, safety,morals, order, peace, comfort, and general welfare of the People" (44, p. 49). Further, states are free to assume responsibility for matters to do with the general welfare not delegated to the federal government under the Constitution, and also may delegate certain responsibilities to local governments. By 1900, some 38 states had public health laws. Laws vary from simply stating broad principles to describing minute details.

Four major roles of the state in matters of health are:
1. Quality control over licensure, vital statistics, medical laborato-

ries, fire and sanitation regulations, OSHA enforcement, and standard setting for preventive health services.

2. Administration of third-party reimbursement programs, especially Medicaid, including priority setting in funding organ transplants.
3. Policy influence on communicable disease control, data collection, and assessment.
4. Delivery of service: maternal/child health care, public health nursing, keeping vital records (Oregon became the first state to list smoking on death certificates [60]), clinic services, laboratory services, health education, mental health care, state hospital care, lead and other kinds of screening (44).
5. Education of the public including environmental health risks.

A study of the public health statutes of the 50 states identified the functions listed in Table 2.3. Each state has a health department,

Table 2.3   State Health Department Functions*

Communicable disease control	Qualifications of local health officers
Sexually transmitted disease control and HIV activities	Chronic disease control
	Milk inspection
Tuberculosis control	Occupational health
Quarantines	Establish/maintain state hospitals
Vital statistics	Children with chronic disabilities
Promulgation of rules and regulations	Health planning
	Housing inspection
Water/stream pollution control	PKU/metabolic screening
	Alcohol, recreational drugs, and addiction control
Facilities inspection	
Facilities licensure	Dental health
Laboratory services	Rabies control
Refuse disposal	Ambulance service
Air pollution control	School health
Abate nuisances/filth	Health personnel registration/ licensure/credentialing
Health education, including communication about environmental risks	Home health care
	Needs and resource assessment
	Nursing care
Radiologic health & disposal of radioactive waste	Family planning
	Extermination services
Food inspection	Compulsory hospitalization
Mental health/illness care	Nutrition programs
Prevention of blindness	Emergency medical services
Maternal/child health	Toxic waste disposal
Immunizations	Caring for deinstitutionalized persons
	Care of indigent and uninsured

*Adapted from Miller et al (9).

funded from state and federal revenues. Generally, there is a state health officer, usually a political appointee, and a state board of health. The board may be composed of physicians or a multidisciplinary group of providers. Consumers may also be represented on it (44). Often board members are political appointees.

In recent times, state influence in health policy making has increased. Some experiments in health care at the state level, such as hospital cost containment, have been the basis for proposals at the federal level. Presently, state government influence over health care is evident in a number of areas:

1. Financing health care for the poor, chronically disabled, and, in some states, those without health insurance.
2. Regulating costs of health care and mandated health benefits for insurers (45).
3. Quality assurance.
4. Education of health care providers.
5. Providing authorization for services of local health authorities (44).

States have also begun to enact statutes supporting death with dignity and the hospice movement. States also have begun to address problems of the uninsured; in 1988, Massachusetts enacted a universal health insurance plan (46). Several others followed that example over the next four years: in 1992, Florida, Minnesota, and Vermont passed legislation aimed at helping those without health insurance or/and to expand Medicaid (39). Hawaii has passed legislation to assure that 98% of its residents are insured. Issues that policy makers in state legislatures will face in the next few years include health planning, the escalation of costs, provision of long-term care, services for an increasing number of elders, services for the mentally disabled, especially as they age, access to prenatal and well child care, regulation of the health insurance industry, AIDS, care of the homeless, and controversies over licensure, credentialing of health care workers, and malpractice issues.

In fiscal 1992, the states projected that they would spend 11.8 billion dollars on health. While federal dollars contributed to state health projects have grown over the last decade, state spending has declined. Other sources, including fee for service, have increased over the same time period. In 1990, expenditures by states included eight percent of their budgets dedicated to health and hospitals (51).

Oregon has led the nation in tackling the problem of limited and declining sources of funding for health care and in prioritizing need. Oregon has been granted an exception to Medicaid rules on mandated coverage to pilot a program to extend Medicaid coverage to all uninsured individuals. In order to do so, however, the legislature has had to make difficult decisions about what benefits will be covered. Nurses have been involved in this experiment from the beginning. Oregon's experiences will be important to consider in any plan for health care reform (58).

The Private Sector

The traditions of American health care are rooted in the private enterprise system. Private independent providers and private hospitals and other institutions comprise a large part of the total system of care. Voluntary private organizations, too, influence health care policy and delivery.

Independent Providers

The largest group of independently practicing providers of health care are physicians. Grounded in the tradition of the first century of American medical practice, these providers have a long heritage of independent practice. From the early 1920s, the American Medical Association has lobbied vigorously to retain control of health care in the private sector (6, pp. 49-59). Private practice is still the dominant model for medical practice in the United States, as it is for others licensed to practice independently (dentists, optometrists, and so on). The majority of physicians are in office practice, although some are still completing their education, some are hospital based, and some are engaged in practices, such as research, that do not involve clients. The majority of physicians in office practice are specialists. In 1990, 88.5% of physicians were in specialty practice (48). Close to

60% of physicians are in office-based practices including solo and group practice and HMOs, or work in industry, insurance companies, health departments, and laboratories. The remainder practice in hospitals, training programs, and work for the federal government (48, p. 108).

Most Americans still receive physician care in the office or in HMOs (48, p. 110). Technology has necessitated the move toward more institutionalization of practice. In fact, the plethora of specialists and the glut of technology mediate for self-diagnosis and confusion on the part of the client experiencing symptoms. Unless the patient has a primary care provider, she/he must often negotiate the maze and try to decide which specialist to call and what services might most appropriately be received. Emphasis on primary care is one attempt to rejuvenate the system and provide for more holistic and sensitive care. If each individual chooses a primary care provider, that provider will act as the coordinator of care and assure the continuity now lacking for so many clients. Primary care also should mean primary prevention (52).

Hospitals

Modern health care technology feeds on a vast array of sophisticated machinery and expert personnel, both of which are found in institutions. Hence, providers and consumers are dependent on these institutions. Dating from the church and monastery-related hostels and hospices of the middle ages, the modern hospital still purports to offer a refuge to the ill. Until the late nineteenth century, however, hospitals were in large part places where one went to die (54).

In 1990, 47.99% of rural and urban hospitals in the United States were private and nonprofit, a change of -3.9% in 10 years. State and local government operated l,444 hospitals in 1990, a change of - 18.8% from 1980-1990. For profit hospitals (N=749) increased in the same decade by 2.6% (48, p. 112). In community hospitals, from 1980-1988, beds increased by 257% and occupancy rates fell from 75.6% to 65.5% (50). In 1990, there were 1,211,000 beds in 6,649 hospitals in the United States. Of these, 928,000 were in community hospitals. Thus, over 69% of all community hospitals were nonprofit.

The bed-per-population ratio should be less than four per thousand, but in 1990, bed ratios were 5.1 per thousand, a change of -15.3% from 1980-1990. For profit beds increased during this period by 16.9%, while long-term general and special beds changed by -36.2%. Federal hospital beds declined 6.1%, a -16.5% change. Unoccupied beds help to escalate health care costs (48).

Hospitals have evolved as relatively independent agencies, historically collaborating little in the total health care efforts. Often governed by a loosely organized structure of trustees, medical staff, and administrators, only in recent years have they begun to be held accountable in a regional sense. With the 1974 National Health Resources and Development Act, the proliferation of the acquisition of technologically sophisticated equipment has slowed, but duplications within geographic areas still occur. The power of the autonomous, independent medical staff may clash with that of administration. Since most clients are admitted by physicians in private practice, hospitals are dependent upon them to keep their beds full. In fact, some would contend that the hospital exists, in large part, as a work place for the physicians (56), a contention they say is borne out by figures on the procedures performed on patients (48). Only in relatively recent years has hospital administration moved into the professional business arena.

The mean occupancy rates for hospitals as of 1988 was below 70% in most of the country and 62.3% in the Midwest, 62% in the South, and 62.4% in the West (50). At the same time, the average number of full-time equivalent employees (FTEs) on any given day in 1988 was 268,000 (50).

There are some similarities between hospitals and hotels. The names come from the same root, the charges are based on daily occupancy, and empty beds mean loss of money (36, p. 77). Perhaps hospital charges should be calculated differently. Rates might vary depending on the amount of care required, the type of diet, and so on. Hotels are much less expensive and may be used in conjunction with hospitals to help keep down the cost of health care. For example, the Children's Inn is adjacent to the Children's Hospital Medical Center in

Boston. The Inn is a hotel where children and their parents stay as an alternative to hospitalization when intensive 24-hour monitoring of care by professionals is not necessary but treatments and assessments are required at intervals (36, p. 262).

Nonfederal long-stay hospitals declined in number from 157 in 1980 to 131 in 1990, and beds decreased from 39,000 to 25,000. Most of the remaining long-term beds are in the 286 state and county government-owned psychiatric facilities, reflecting a move toward more outpatient care and deinstitutionalization (50).

Nursing Homes

It is a fairly recent phenomenon in this country that nursing homes are run for profit. Less than 50 years ago most nursing homes were sponsored by local governments, churches, or fraternal organizations. With a sharp increase in the number of elders there has come a corresponding increase in nursing homes (48).

The nursing home industry is a large and profitable one. Two modern developments are the nursing home corporations, into which the public may buy stock, and nursing home chains. This industry has been marketed by owners whose primary interest is profit at the expense of the residents.

By 1986, the majority of nursing homes were run for profit. Of the 25,646 in the country, 20,223 were proprietary, and about 90% of the total was certified for Medicare or Medicaid. Since 1963, nursing home beds have increased dramatically (48). The percentage of elderly in nursing homes has continued to increase and the use of nursing homes in this country is higher than in certain other industrialized countries (48). Future health care policy makers will need to examine the nursing home model as to its efficacy and sensitivity in providing care for older Americans.

Voluntary Agencies

Voluntary health agencies, now numbering more than 100,000, were begun in 1892 with the Anti-Tuberculosis Society in Philadelphia (44,

p. 51). They may be loosely divided into three categories: those concerned with specific organs or structures such as the heart, lungs, or eyes; those concerned with specific diseases such as tuberculosis or cancer; and those that concern themselves with the general welfare of special groups, such as children, adults of childbearing age, or the elderly (44, p. 55). In 1989, voluntary health agencies raised about one billion dollars, 481 million from corporations (48). Most of it was raised by about two dozen of the largest agencies, including the American Cancer Society, Inc., The American Heart Association, The American Lung Association, the National Foundation March of Dimes, and the National Easter Seal Society for Crippled Adults and Children. Of American households, 32.4% gave to health-related charities an average of $143.00 (48).

Although the total of all the voluntary agency budgets is but a small fraction of the federal budget for health, the impact of these agencies on health education and information is enormous (59). They must, therefore, be viewed as an important and significant part of the private sector of our health care delivery system.

Summary

The roles of government and the private sector in the total scheme of our health care delivery system are inextricably interwoven. Increases in federal spending for health over the past few years have markedly increased the interrelationship. The following chapters will explore some of the subsystems in more depth and suggest paths we may follow in years to come. Whatever paths we tread, it is likely that we will continue to have important input from both sectors.

References

1. Dolan, J.A. (1978). Nursing in Society. 14th ed. Philadelphia: Saunders.
2. Walsh, M.R. (1977). Doctors Wanted: No Women Need Apply. New Haven: Yale University Press, p. 5.

3. Dock, L.L. and Steward, I.M. (1936). A Short History of Nursing. 4th ed. New York: Putnam's Sons.

4. Kaufman, M. (1976). American Medical Education: The Formative Years, 1765-1910. Westport, CT: Greenwood Press.

5. Dietz, L.D. (1963). History and Modern Nursing. Philadelphia: F.A. Davis, p. 94.

6. Cray, E. (1970). In Failing Health. Indianapolis: Bobbs-Merrill.

7. Miller, C.A., Gilbert, B., Warren, D.C., Brooks, E.F., DeFriese, G.H., Jain, S.C. and Kavaler, F. (1977). Statutory authorizations for the work of local health departments. American Journal of Public Health 67(10):940-945.

8. Programs of HUD. (1992). Washington, DC: U.S. Department of Housing and Urban Development.

9. Miller, C.A., Brooks, E.F., DeFriese, G.H., Gilbert, B., Jain, S.C., and Kavaler, F. (1977). A survey of local public health departments and their directors. American Journal of Public Health 67(10):931-939.

10. News. (October 1992). United States Department of Agriculture, Food and Nutrition Service.

11. Jonas, S., Banta, D. (1986). Government in the health care delivery system. In: S. Jonas, ed., Health Care Delivery in the United States. 3rd ed. New York: Springer.

12. Facts About the Food Programs of the U.S. Department of Agriculture. (1983). Washington, DC: Department of Agriculture.

13. Supplemental Food Programs of the United States Department of Agriculture. (1981). Washington, DC: Department of Agriculture.

14. United States Department of Agriculture Organizational Chart. (1980). Washington, DC: Department of Agriculture.

15. U.S. Department of Labor Program Highlights. (1988). Fact Sheet No. OIPA 88-3.

16. United States Department of Labor. (1990). Fact Sheet No. OIPA 90-1.

17. Major Laws Administered by the U.S. Department of Labor Which Affect Small Business. (1989). Boston: U.S. Department of Labor Region I.

18. U.S. Department of Labor. (1991). Washington, DC: U. S.Department of Labor.

18a. DeFriese, G.H., Hetherington, J.S., Brooks, E.F., Miller, C.A., Jain, S.C., Kasaler, F., and Stein, J.S. (1981). The program implications of administrative relationships between local health departments and state and local government. American Journal of Public Health 71(10):1109-1115.

18b. Jain, S.C., ed. (1981). Role of state and local governments in relation to personal health services. American Journal of Public Health 71(15) (entire issue).

18c. Rohrer, H.H. and Dellaportas, G. (1982). Trends and patterns in characteristics of local health administrators. American Journal of Public

Health 72(8):846-849.

19. Forness, N.O. (1976). Creation of the Department of the Interior, March 3, 1849. Washington, DC: Department of the Interior, Office of Communications, p.3.

20. America's Guardian of Natural Resources. (1978). U.S. Department of Interior Pub. No. 0-275-481. Washington, DC: Government Printing Office.

21. Bureau of Justice Assistance Fact Sheet. (1992). Washington, DC: U.S. Department of Justice.

22. Counting for Representation: The Census and the Constitution. (1990). Washington, DC: U.S. Department of Commerce, Bureau of the Census.

23. Department of Energy. (1991). Washington, DC: The United States Government Manual 1991/92, pp. 273-283.

24. The John A. Volpe National Transportation Systems Center. (1991). Cambridge, MA: Research and Programs Administration, U.S. Department of Transportation.

25. Special Agents. (1988). Washington, DC: U.S. Department of the Treasury, Bureau of Alcohol, Tobacco and Firearms.

26. Welcome to the Department of Education. (1988). Washington, DC: U.S. Department of Education.

27. ACTION Fact Sheet. (1988). Washington, DC: ACTION News.

28. Kirschstein, R.L. (1991). Research on women's health. American Journal of Public Health 81(3):291-293.

29. Federal Physicians Go Everywhere...A Guide to Medical Activities and Organizations of the Federal Government. (1988). Washington, DC: The U.S. Medicine Guide, 1988.

30. Morbidity and Mortality Weekly Report. (1992). 41(44):833.

31. Special Report: FDA. (1988). West Point, PA: Merck & Company.

32. U.S. Public Health Service Recruitment. (undated).

33. Pennock, M.R. (ed.) (1928). Makers of Nursing History. New York: Lakeside, p. 74.

34. Division of Nursing. Hyattsville, MD: U.S. Department of Health, Education, and Welfare, Pub. No. HRA-78-57.

35. Practice Nursing on the Leading Edge. (1989). Washington, DC: U.S. Department of Health and Human Services.

36. Freymann, J.G. (1974). The American Health Care System: Its Genesis and Trajectory. New York: MEDCOM Press.

37. American Red Cross. (1961). Clara Barton: Heroic Woman. Washington, DC: The American National Red Cross.

38. American Red Cross. (1972). Jane Delano: Innovator in Nursing. Washington, DC: The American National Red Cross.

39. State health reports. (1992). The Nation's Health 22(7):17.

40. Chess, C., Salomone, K.L., and Sandman, P.M. (1991). Risk commu-

nication activities of state health agencies. American Journal of Public Health 81(4):489-491.

41. Duffy, J. (1966). Sword of Pestilence. Baton Rouge: Louisiana State University Press, p. 145.

42. Rosen, G. (1958). A History of Public Health. New York: M.D. Publications, p. 234.

43. Merritt, R. (1988). Oregon transplant policy provokes prevention vs. high-tech controversy. The Nation's Health 18(3):20.

44. Role of state and local governments in relation to personal health services. (1981). American Journal of Public Health 71, January (entire issue).

45. States move more cautiously on mandated health benefits. (1987). The Nation's Health 17(10-11):12.

46. Massachusetts passes state health insurance. (1988). The Nation's Health 18(5-6):1-3.

47. Preserving the Future. Your Guide to the United States Environmental Protection Agency. (1991). Washington, DC: Communications and Public Affairs, EPA.

48. Statistical Abstract of the United States 1992. (1992). 112th ed. Washington, DC: U.S. Department of Commerce, Bureau of the Census.

49. National Center for Health Statistics. (1988). Hyettsville, MD: National Center for Health Statistics.

50. State and Metropolitan Area Data Book 1991. (1991). Washington, DC: Department of Commerce, Economics and Statistics Administration.

51. Budget woes force SHAS to make cuts. (1992). Public Health Macroview 5(1):1-3.

52. Milio, N. (1983). Primary Care and the Public Health. Lexington, MA: D.C. Heath.

53. Capuzzi, C. and Garland, M. (1990). The Oregon plan: Increasing access to health care. Nursing Outlook 38(6):260-263,286.

54. Somers, A.R. and Somers, H.M. (1977). Health and Health Care. Germantown, MD: Aspen Systems, p. 85.

55. Milio, N. (1975). The Care of Health in Communities. Access for Outcasts. New York: Macmillan, pp. 85-86.

56. Ginzberg, E. (1969). Men, Money, and Medicine. New York: Columbia University Press, p. 91.

57. Health in the United States. Chartbook. (1980). Washington, DC: U.S. Department of Health, Education, and Welfare, Public Health Service, Office of Health Research, Statistics, and Technology.

58. Fisher, E.S., Welch, H.G., & Wennberg, J.E. (1992). Prioitizing Oregon's hospital resources. Journal of the American Medical Association 267(14):1925-1931.

59. Voluntary health agencies: Small sums, strong voices. (1978). The

Nation's Health 8(6):7,12.
60. Oregon death certificates to list smoking. (1988). The New York Times, Sept. 1, B14.
61. Pickett, G. (1989). Local public health and the state. American Journal of Public Health 79(8):967-968.
62. Shea, S. (1992). Community health, community risks, community action. American Journal of Public Health 82(6):785-787.
63. Flynn, B.C. and Rider, M.S. (1991). Healthy cities, Indiana: Mainstreaming community health in the United States. American Journal of Public Health 81(4):510-511.
64. Jurs, J. (1991). The role of the local health department in traffic safety. American Journal of Public Health 81(4):511-512.
65. Spain, C., Eastman, E., and Kizer, K.W. (1989). Model standards impact on local health department performance in California. American Journal of Public Health 79(8):969-974.
66. Adams-Ender, C.L., Jennings, B., Bartz, C., and Jensen, R. (1991). Nursing practice models: The Army Nurse Crops Experience. Nursing and Health Care 12(3):120-123.
67. Baker, E. L. (ed.) (1989). Surveillance in occupational health and safety. American Journal of Public Health 79 (Supp.).
68. VA Today. (1989). Washington, DC: Department of Veterans Affairs.
69. The National Health Service Corps Summary Fact Sheet, 1992.
70. Agency for Health Care Policy and Research, 1989. Unpublished Highlight Summary, PL 101-239.
71. Mercer, M.E. (1992). News about the restructuring of ADAMHA: Center for Mental Health Services. ANA Council Perspectives 1(3)2.

3

Federal Health Care Legislation

Federal legislation concerned with health dates to the 1798 bill which established the United States Marine Hospital Service for Sick and Disabled Seamen (1,p.44). That bill marked the beginning of nearly two centuries of accelerating federal legislation for health. In this chapter, we will look as some of the major pieces of legislation passed during those years and at the current proposals for health care reform. In order to provide a framework for those discussions, however, the first section will deal with the legislative process and with how nurses, as providers and consumers, can influence and be a part of that process.

The Legislative Process

The legislative branch of our federal government is, of course, responsible for passing the bills which provide for health and welfare programs for the nation's citizens. The process of passing a bill such as the Nurse Training Act of 1971 or the Rural Health Clinics Services Act of 1978 is complex and involves far more than introducing the bill to the Senate and the House of Representatives and obtaining a vote. Our Congressmen and women spend most of their working time in the Senate and

House office buildings rather than in the Senate and House chambers. The House and Senate have standing or legislative committees, as well as conference, select (ad hoc), and joint committees. The number of these will vary in each branch of Congress and from one session of Congress to another. Members and chairpersons of these committees wield a great deal of power. Special committees may also be called as needed to investigate concerns and hold hearings. Only the standing committees can report bills to the floor of the House or Senate, however (2).

A bill begins its life when a draft of it is placed in the "hopper," a large box on the floor of each of the houses of Congress. This draft may vary from a few words to a formal document of substantial length. After the bill is introduced, it is referred to the appropriate committee(s) and then to the appropriate subcommittee(s) where it either dies a quiet death or is considered. If it is a bill of importance, public hearings will be held at which representatives of the administration and the public may air their views. It is at this point that mailgrams, letters, postcards, night letters, faxes, telephone calls, personal visits, and public opinion telegrams can be helpful in influencing the process.

After the hearings, if the bill is still considered to be significant, a final draft is hammered out in subcommittee(s) at what is known as a "mark-up session" and then is voted to go to the full committee(s). The full committee(s) will review it and may hold more hearings. A majority vote sends it to the floor of the House or Senate. It is then assigned a number preceded by "H. Res." or "S. Res." (House Resolution or Senate Resolution), "H. J. Res." or "Sen. J. Res." (House Joint Resolution or Senate Joint Resolution), or "H. Con. Res." or "S. Con. Res." (House Concurrent Resolution or Senate Concurrent Resolution).

Before a bill goes to the House floor for a vote, the Rules Committee reviews it and decides if amendments are appropriate and, if so, in what form a debate about them may take place and how long the debate can be. The Rules Committee can also delay or kill a bill. The Senate does not have a Rules Committee (2).

Floor action begins with the introduction of the bill by the committee chairperson. Debate may last minutes or days. Once the work on a bill is completed by one body, the other body begins, or the two houses may work on the same bill simultaneously. Sometimes a bill is killed because the House-Senate conference committee cannot agree. After the conference committee meets, both houses must pass a final, identical version of the bill. Then it goes to the President for a signature. If the President vetoes it, Congress can override the veto by a two-thirds vote of both houses (2).

In order for monies to be appropriated for a program, Congress must first pass a bill authorizing the federal government to operate the program. Then an appropriations bill must be passed to allow the money to be spent. Congress, however, must pass these requests within 45 days. The President has the authority to defer spending the money by a deferral decision, or he can rescind the money so that it will not be spent (2).

Virtually all the committees of the House and Senate can deal with bills that directly or indirectly affect the health of the nation's citizens. The Finance and Appropriations Committees of the Senate, and the Budget, Ways and Means, and Appropriations Committees of the House, are directly involved in funding for federal dollars spent on health care.

Legislative processes are affected by a number of factors including the political ramifications of the issues,   career aspirations of chairpersons and members of committees, the sensitivity of committee members to pressures from the administration, lobbying groups, the members' party leadership and affiliations, the pet interests of members, and the legislative calendar for that session (3).

Nursing's Role in the Process

The American Nurses Association is now headquartered in Washington, DC, where it maintains a lobbying presence with a full-time staff. Most of their time is spent in gathering information in order to present the most positive and accurate view of nursing. The association's representatives also inform members of Congress about nursing affairs either directly or through Congressional staff members. In addition, the association's staff members help educate nurses about bills affecting health care and nursing (4). Representatives from nursing across the nation may go to Washington to testify before committees, to attend critical meetings, and to call on members of Congress or the administration. The Association's staff help to coordinate such efforts.

There are those who are highly critical of the lobbying roles played by professional organizations. For example, when the American Nurses' Association lobbies to legislate 24-hour registered nurse coverage in nursing homes, these critics may ask whether this is for the good of the patients or for the good of nursing as a profession. Feldstein, a health economist, has argued that professional organizations' positions on proposed health legislation "will be based upon its perceived effect on the membership's interests, though this position is often presented as being in the best interests of the public." (5, p. 5) This is a serious charge and an issue that nurses must weigh carefully. Although there are many instances when what is good for patients is also good for nursing, it is all too easy for an organization to become self-serving. We must continually question our own motives and priorities.

Over a number of years, the Robert Wood Johnson Foundation (private) and the Kellogg Foundation have funded health policy fellowships in Washington, DC, for nurses, as do several other private foundations and educational groups (10). Some of these nurses have helped to draft the American Nurses Association's positions on health matters. Sister Donley reports from her experiences in Washington that constituents have a tremendous impact on those who represent them in Congress. A favorite ploy of congresspeople is to begin a speech in committee or on the House floor with a tale from a constituent (3).

Other sources of public policy fellowships for which nurses can apply include the President's Commission on White House Fellowships, Congressional Fellowships on Women and Public Policy, the Congressional Research Grants Program, the Judicial Fellowship Program, and the Office of Technology Assessment Congressional Fellowship Program (10).

The Nurses' Coalition for Action in Politics (N-CAP), founded in 1974, is dedicated to improving health care through the political process. It attempts to accomplish this through educating nurses about the political process, encouraging them to get involved, and raising funds to support candidates who show concern for issues related to nursing and health care. Now called ANA-PAC, it exists as the political arm of the ANA, but is separately organized with its own trustees.

ANA-PAC is active at the national level, but there are also political action committees (PACs) for state-level political action. Nurses in some 38 states in 1984 had such committees. Nineteen seventy-six was the first year in which ANA endorsed candidates (6). Criteria for backing candidates are based on the health policy positions and legislative priorities of the American Nurses Association. ANA reviews every congressional race and, in consultation with its PACs in those states in which they exist, evaluates candidates. American Nurses Association congressional lobbyists in Washington review candidates and check voting records of incumbents on health and nursing issues. Then the ANA-PAC screening committee makes recommendations to the trustees who make the decisions about whom to support. State nurses' associations and state PACs are notified of these decisions as are the candidates (7).

Specialty nursing organizations have organized the Nurses' Coalition for Legislative Action to work at the federal level for those organizations. This coalition will help to create a united voice for the profession from the dozens of nursing organizations (7).

PACs have come under considerable criticism recently because the large amounts of money they command enable them to wield considerable influence. Some candidates for political office have declared that they will not accept money from PACs in order to disassociate themselves from influence by those groups (2).

How to Analyze Legislation

A very important role we can assume in the legislative process at the local, state, and federal level is analyzing proposed legislation. With our knowledge of the effects of health care legislation on our patients, their families, significant others, and communities, we bring a unique perspective from which to analyze legislation that will result in health policy (9). Analysis of proposed legislation or public policy allows us to direct our efforts most effectively in influencing the course of a piece of legislation or the outcome of efforts to create or change public policy.

In analyzing a piece of legislation, there are several questions we can ask that will help us determine whether or not it will accomplish what the bill intends and in which direction our lobbying activities should be focused. In Table 3.1, there is a list of suggested questions to guide our analysis.

Positing our analysis within an ethical framework is one perspective that we can adopt. The Cabinet on Ethics of one state nurses association developed guidelines for nurses to analyze policies that may affect the health and well being of the public. These guidelines appear as Table 3.2.

Table 3.1   Questions to Ask in Analyzing Health Care Legislation Affecting Health Care

---

- Whom will it serve and who is covered?
- Who will pay for what the bill is proposing?
- Will it raise or lower costs?
- Does it assure access to providers?
- What actual amount of money will be used for direct care versus bureaucratic costs?
- What services will be paid for? Is it a deductible plan? Are there limits to coverage or coinsurance?
- Who will profit or benefit?
- Education bills—who gets the money? Students? Schools? What are the restrictions on use?
- Does the bill propose new programs or support or supplement those already in existence?
- If the bill deals with support for nursing research, who can apply? To whom will the money go?

Table 3.2 Moral Dimensions of Public Policy Formation: Guidelines for Nurses*

The United States health care system has experienced unprecedented growth in the past four decades. With this growth in scientific knowledge, advanced technology and increased cost, the role of public policy has become one of primary importance. Citizens expect their federal, state, and local government to formulate coherent health care policies to meet the needs of society. The nursing profession has made a commitment to provide health care services to society [1]; each nurse has an obligation to be an active participant in the public policy process. Public policies are multidimensional, incorporating legal, economic, organizational, political, scientific/technological, and ethical dimensions [2]. Recognizing the complexity of the public policy process, the Massachusetts Nurses Association (MNA) Cabinet on Ethics has developed these guidelines to assist nurses in the assessment of public policies from an ethical perspective.

Nurses are guided in their practice by a Code of Ethics reflecting the moral principles and values held by their profession [3]. Their obligation to particpate in the public policy process is twofold: first, to help make and shape policies which wil enhance the general health and welfare of the people they serve; second, to perserve the moral principles and values of the nursing profession and society.

Operating Principles

1. An operating principle of nursing is respect for the inherent dignity and equal worth of every person [4]. Public policies must reflect adherence to this principle.

2. The nurse's primary commitment is the health, welfare and safety of the client. Nevertheless, public policies relating to health care must reflect a just balance between the rights of the individual and the rights of society.

3. The terms **benefits** and **burdens** are used in the assessment of the allocation and distribution of both social benefits (goods and services, such as health care) and social burdens (taxation and suffering experienced by denial of goods and services).

Public Policy: Definition and Process

"Public policies are defined as those policies developed by officials and government bodies which determine a course of action for dealing with a problem or matter of public concern [5]." The seven stages in the process of public policy formation are:

Stage 1: Policy Formation
The government acknowledges the problem.

Stage 2: Policy Agenda
The government initiates debate on the problem.

Stage 3: Policy Formulation
The government proposes solutions to the problem.

Stage 4: Policy Analysis
The government examines alternative solutions and options.

Stage 5: Policy Adoption
The government adopts a particular solution to the problem.

Stage 6: Policy Implementation
The government applies its resources to the problem.

State 7: Policy Evaluation
The government evaluates the effectiveness of the policy in achievement of its goals [6].

Questions to Assist Nurses in Assessing the Moral Dimensions of Public Policies

The process of assessing a policy from an ethical dimension requires asking questions that address the moral dimensions of the policy throughout the seven stages. The following is a comprehensive, but not all-inclusive, list of questions to consider:

1. What is the purpose of this policy?
2. Who wrote/proposed this policy?
3. Who are the target populations?

(Continued)

Table 3.2 (Continued)

4. How does this policy benefit the target populations?
5. What groups are included and what groups are excluded in this policy?
6. Are there equal benefits and burdens to all people affected by this policy?
7. Are the rights of one group denied in order to promote the rights of another group?
8. What are the origin and adequacy of the resources needed to implement this policy?
9. Will the resources be justly allocated; that is, will they be allocated on the basis of the equal worth of all human beings?
10. Are there alternatives which would be more equitable?

escalating costs of acute care impair our ability to provide preventive and chronic care?

Nurses must view proposed public policies relating to health care from a societal context as opposed to only looking at the needs of a specific population. Implementation of these guidelines will inform nurses' decision making in assessing public policies and strengthen their role as advocates for a just system of health care. As the nation's policies reflect its values, so too, must nursing's visions reflect the profession's commitment to the health of all people.

Conclusions

The impact of public policies on nursing's ability to deliver health care fairly to all persons is illustrated in the issue of allocation of resources for health care on the federal, state, and local levels. As government strives to meet the competing claims of various groups within society, nursing is faced with the problem of meeting the health care needs of individuals from diverse populations. When are resources taken from one group to meet the needs of another? For example, in meeting the health care needs of the fast growing population of elders, can we compromise the health care needs of the young? Will the

References

Footnotes
1. *Nursing: A Social Policy Statement*, American Nurses' Association, Kansas City, MO, 1980.
2. Carroll, James D., *Dimensions of Public Policy*. Brookings Institution, Washington D.C. Unpublished Manuscript.
3. American Nurses' Association *Code for Nurses with Interpretive Statements*, American Nurses' Association, Kansas City, MO, 1985.
4. Ibid.
5. Sisters of Mercy Health Corporation, *Health Services for the Poor: A Challenge to Public Policy*, Sisters of Mercy Health Corporation. Farmington Hills, Michigan, 1985, p. 1.
6. Anderson, F., et al, *Public Policy and Politics in America*, second edition. Monterey, California, Brooks-Cole Publishing Company, 1978.

* Cabinet on Nursing Ethics, Massachusetts Nurses Association. Used with permission.

How to Influence Legislation

First of all, it is important to keep well informed. There are many sources of information about bills being considered in the committees and subcommittees of the Senate and House. *The American Nurse* (ANA's official newspaper), *The Nation's Health* (the American Public Health Association's newspaper), *The American Journal of Nursing,* and publications of the National League for Nursing are all invaluable sources. The local offices of senators and representatives can provide materials about bills. You can request inclusion of your name on their mailing lists. In a presidential election year, the local offices of the major parties will readily supply material on their candidates. Copies

Table 3.3   Sources of Information on Legislation

Information	Source
General information, updates of legislation; Congressional action	*The Nation's Health* American Public Health Association 1015 18th Street, N.W. Washington, D.C. 20036 Subscriptions available to nonmembers
	The American Nurse American Nurses Association 600 Maryland Ave. SW, Suite 100 West Washington, D.C. 20024-2571 Subscriptions available to nonmembers
	Congressional Record Superintendent of Documents Government Printing Office, Washington, D.C. 20402
	Federal Register Office of Federal Register National Archives and Record Service Washington, D.C. 20408
Copies of bills, amendments, public laws (free to press, government officials, college libraries, faculty, students, nonprofit organizations)	Newsletters of organizations in a particular field, state and local agencies Appropriate offices such as Aged, Children, and Youth Send number and title of bill you wish to: Senate Document Room U.S. Capitol S-3211 Washington, D.C. 20510 OR House Document Room U.S. Capitol H-226 Washington, D.C. 20515
Committee Reports	Write to appropriate committee U.S. Senate, Washington, D.C. 20510 OR U.S. House of Representatives Washington, D.C. 20515
GAO Reports	Distribution Section General Accounting Office 441 G. Street, N.W., Room 4522 Washington, D.C. 20548

of the party platforms are available after the national conventions from local or state party offices.

The Congressional Record, the official record of the proceedings and debates of Congress, will help to keep you informed of the course of a piece of legislation. Your local librarian can tell you where the repository of government documents is for your area. Copies of bills can be obtained through the sponsoring or administering government department (such as Health and Human Services), and many materials explaining programs and legislation are available through the U.S. Government Printing Office, Superintendent of Documents, Washington, DC, 20402 (see Table 3.3).

In order to influence your senators and representatives, write letters or send postcards, telegraphs, public opinion telegrams (limited to 20 words), faxes, mailgrams, or nightletters. Make letters short, succinct, and reflective of your position or the position you wish your representative to take. It is also good to include any pertinent information you might have to back your position. Our representatives cannot be fully knowledgeable about the hundreds of bills they are expected to vote on, and they are usually glad to receive material which increases their understanding. Be sure you are well informed about the contents of the bill you are writing about (see Table 3.4 for how to address letters).

Going to Washington to lobby or testify for or against a bill is a way to become politically involved. Washington professionals expect you to be knowledgeable, accurate, and honest in representing your position, and also succinct since time is valuable. Interpersonal skills acquired through nursing should serve you well (2, 8). It is usually possible to see your representative in person with a prior appointment. Senate interviews are usually carried out by staff members. Know your purpose so you can convey it quickly and in a well-informed way. Let your legislator know whether you want him or her to introduce or support a bill or amendment, or whether you want testimony on a bill that has been introduced. Your members of Congress can also help you locate the right office or person within the Department of Health and Human Services if you need information (3).

Table 3.4   How to Address Senators and Representatives

The Honorable Senator _____
Dirksen OR Russell Senate Office Building
Washington, D.C. 20510

Dear Senator _____ :

The Honorable Congressman (woman) _____
Cannon House Office Building
OR
Longworth House Office Building
OR
Rayburn House Office Building
Washington, D.C. 20515

Dear Congressman (woman) _____:

Another way to be involved in political and legislative processes is to support candidates for office. Check the candidate out for issues you are concerned about. ANA-PAC can help you learn about candidates for national offices, and state PACs and/or local party offices will help you with information about candidates for state and local offices. Your support can range from donations to making calls, helping with mailings, hosting neighborhood meetings, and doing door-to-door promotion. You could advise candidates on health issues and health legislation (2).

Voting is an essential contribution to the political and legislative process. Be sure to register. Your county courthouse, state election office, or city clerk can tell you how and where; procedures vary from town to town and state to state. You can also participate by urging others to register and to vote. Within nursing, you can encourage your colleagues to register and vote (7).

On the state level, information about health related legislation can be gleaned from your state nurses' association and from the offices of your state senator and representative. Often the state or local League of Women Voters puts out an information bulletin on the legislature or general assembly, so they are worth contacting. Some states have a bill information retrieval service which operates through the state library system. Your local librarian could help you obtain this service if it is available. It is possible to attend public hearings and to lobby for bills at the state level in a manner similar to that at the national level.

Town and county political structures vary across the nation. Your local town or county office can inform you of the decision-making structure in your area and how you can become involved.

Health Care Legislation

The saga of the development of legislation concerning health is a fascinating one. The first bill, passed by Congress in 1798, started the steady evolution of federal involvement in health care policy and delivery of health services. (See Table 3.5) Throughout the nineteenth century, federal involvement with health care might be characterized as a congenial but distant interest. Bills to increase the responsibilities of the Marine Hospital Service, to charge the Department of War and then the Department of the Interior with Indian health affairs, to provide monies to support mental hospitals and to aid deaf-mutes and the blind, and to administer Freedman's and St. Elizabeth's Hospitals were passed (1, pp. 44-45).

The American Medical Association, informally organized in 1847, supported increased federal involvement in health care, specifically the creation of a federal health department with cabinet-level status (1, p. 47). Interestingly, it was not until 1953 that such an act was passed, creating the Department of Health, Education, and Welfare. In 1906, the Pure Food and Drugs Act was passed with American Medical Association support (1, p. 48). The Children's Bureau was created in 1912, the same year in which the Public Health Service was given its present name. In 1922, a bill was passed to provide monies for child health care. Child and maternity centers established under that bill existed until 1929, when Congress failed to appropriate more monies for

Table 3.5	Major U.S. Federal Legislation and Administrative Activities Related to Health*

1798	Bill to create the United States Marine Hospital Service (MHS) for Sick and Disabled Seamen.
1849	Indian Health Affairs assigned to Department of Interior.
1854	Congress allocated 10 million acres in each state, income from which was to support mental hospitals; 2.5 million acres in each state to support deaf mutes and the blind.
1870	Reorganization of Marine Hospital Service on national basis.
1884	Financing of Marine Hospital Service through tax levied on merchant marine tonnage.
1893	Marine Hospital Service charged by Congress to be responsible for all foreign and interstate quarantine.
1905	Marine Hospital Service funded through general tax fund.
1906	Pure Food and Drugs Act.
1912	Creation of Children's Bureau; Marine Hospital Service renamed Public Health Service.
1922	Bill to provide monies for child health care and establish child and maternity centers.
1935	Social Security Act.
1944	Public Health Service Act extended to all National Institutes of Health the authority to award research grants to non-federal establishments.
1946	Hill-Burton legislation authorizing federal assistance in the construction of hospitals and health centers; to improve population bed ratios, especially in rural areas. National Mental Health Act — National Institute of Mental Health created.
1948	Creation of the National Heart Institute and the National Institute of Dental Research as part of a broadened National Institutes of Health.
1949	Establishment of a common system of ten regional offices of the Federal Security Agency (later to become the nucleus of the Department of Health, Education, and Welfare).
1950	Amendments to Social Security Act — allowed payments to vendors for medical services and for old age assistance payments to persons in public medical institutions.
1953	Establishment of the Department of Health, Education, and Welfare as a cabinet-status agency.
1956	Authorization of the National Health Survey, a continuing interview and clinical appraisal of the health of Americans.

Table 3.5 (Continued)

Establishment of the National Library of Medicine.

1958 Amendments to the 1906 Food, Drug, and Cosmetic Act requiring manufacturers of new food additives to submit evidence to the Food and Drug Administration that a product's safety had been tested and established before marketing.

1960 Kerr-Mills Bill giving federal aid to states to cover part of costs of medical services to indigent aged.

Establishment of the Division of Air Pollution in the Public Health Service.

1962 Organization of a Special Staff on Aging, later to become the Administration on Aging.

1963 Health Professions Educational Assistance Act to help meet critical manpower shortages:

The Mental Retardation Facilities and Community Mental Health Centers Construction Act.

Clean Air Act giving assistance to state and local governments to meet the problems of air pollution.

1964 Nurse Training Act, aiding construction of new schools for nursing students and support for curriculum development.

Economic Opportunity Act, creating the Office of Economic Opportunity (OEO).

Hospital and Medical Facilities amendments to Hill-Burton Act allowed for more construction and renovation and for neighborhood health centers and emergency room facilities.

Civil Rights Act.

1965 Establishment of the Federal Water Pollution Control Administration.

Establishment of the National Clearinghouse for Smoking and Health.

Medicare—medical health insurance for citizens 65 and over.

Medicaid—medical assistance program for the indigent.

Regional Medical Programs Act—regional cooperation in health care planning.

Drug Abuse Control Amendments.

Cigarette Labeling and Advertising Act.

Mental Retardation Facilities and Community Mental Health Centers Construction Act amendments.

Community Health Centers Extension amendments.

Health Research Facilities amendments.

Water Quality Act.

Clean Air Act Amendments.

Health Professions Educational Assistance Amendments.

Medical Library Assistance Act.

Table 3.5 (Continued)

Appalachian Regional Development Act.
Older Americans Act.
Solid Waste Disposal Act.
Vocational Rehabilitation Act amendments.
Housing and Urban Development Act.

1966- Public Health Service Act amendments — monies for planning
1967   health care.

1967   Clinical Laboratories Improvement Act authorizing establish-
       ment of minimum performance standards for all clinical
       laboratories engaged in interstate commerce.

1968   Vocational Rehabilitation amendments extending appropria-
       tions for grants to states for services, innovation projects,
       and training.
       Health Manpower Act — monies for schools of nursing.

1969   Establishment of the National Center for Family Planning.

1970   Migrant Health Amendments extended health services for
       migrant and other seasonal agricultural workers.
       Creation of the Environmental Protection Agency.
       National Institute on Alcohol Abuse and Alcoholism and the
       National Institute on Drug Abuse.
       Occupational Safety and Health Act (administered prin-
       cipally by the Department of Labor) to regulate and cor-
       rect health hazards of the workplace.

1971   National Cancer Act.
       Nurse Training Act — capitation grants to schools; support
       for advanced education.
       First federal law to reduce hazard of lead poisoning in
       children.

1972   Social Security Act Amendments: - creating PSRO; further
       defined benefits under Medicaid and Medicare; impor-
       tant new benefits include dialysis.
       National Sickle Cell Anemia Control Act
       National Multiple Sclerosis Act.

1973   HMO Act — model for development of HMO's and funds for
       demonstration projects.

1974   Sudden Infant Death Syndrome Act.
       National Diabetes Mellitus Act.
       National Health Planning and Resource Development Act.

1975   National Arthritis Act.
       Community Mental Health Centers amendments stressing
       services for children, the elderly, rape victims, and
       alcohol and drug abusers.

1976   National Health Consumer and Health Promotion Act.
       Establishment of the Office of Health Information.

Table 3.5 (Continued)

1977 Rural Health Clinic Services Act.

1979 Nurse Training amendments.
Bill to create Department of Education (cabinet level) and
rename Health, Education and Welfare, the Department of
Health and Human Services.

1981 Omnibus Budget Reconciliation Act (P.L. 97-35) created block
grants for maternal child health, prevention programs, TB
programs, alcohol, drug and mental health programs, primary
care, and programs for older adults.

1982 Home Health Training Grant Program.

1983 Amendments to the Social Security Act (P.L. 98-21)
establishing prospective payment under Medicare using
DRGs.

Community Nursing Centers Legislation introduced in the
Senate (S 410) and in the House (HR 4865—1984) for support
of nursing centers through direct third party
reimbursement.

1984 Cost containment Plan (all payer) for hospital and physician
prospective payment introduced.

NIH reauthorization bill introduced to establish an Institute
for Arthritis, Musculoskeletal and Skin Disease.

Reauthorization of Nurse Training Act through fiscal 1987.

Act to provide government assistance to local organ
transplant activities.

Legislation to improve efforts to evaluate existing and new
medical technologies.

Child abuse protection bill including protection under a
Baby Doe clause (withholding treatment can constitute
abuse).

1985 Health Research Extension Act authorizing creation of the
National Center for Nursing Research under N.I.H.

1986 Bill allowing certified registered nurse anesthetists to bill
Medicare directly starting Jan. 1, 1989; risk retention act
allowing groups such as certified nurse midwives with
similar interest to form a self-insurance pool.

Health Care Quality Improvement Act; provisions for peer review
activities and reporting mechanism for malpractice claims and
disciplinary actions against licensed health care professionals.

1986 Public Law 99-272, Title X of the Congressional Omnibus Budget
Reconciliation Act (COBRA) requires that most employers with group
health plans offer continuation coverage for 18 months after
eligibility for the group plan ends.

Table 3.5 (Continued)

1987   Older Americans Act Amendments—four-year reauthorization of
       programs under OAA.
       National health Service Corps authorization extended.
       Medicaid amendments to increase coverage to poor pregnant women
       and children to age 1, eligible with incomes at 185% of
       federal poverty level.

1988   Extension of the National Health Service Corps scholarship program
       as well as authorizing medical school loan repayments to attract
       physicians to the Corps and to work on Indian reservations.
       Catastrophic health insurance legislation under Medicare.
       Nursing shortage reduction and education act.
       AIDS counseling and testing act and AIDS research act.
       Abandoned infants assistance act.

1988   Pepper long-term home care bill.
       Veterans' Benefits and Services Act.
       Qualified Medicare Beneficiary program allows poor seniors and
       persons with disabilities to avoid out-of-pocket payments under
       Medicare.
       HMO Act amendments rewritten.
       Clinical Laboratory Act regulating personnel training and workload.
       Medicare Catastrophic Protection Act.
       Anti-Drug Abuse Act—created Office of National Drug Control Policy
       in the Executive Office of the President.

1989   Rural Nursing Incentive Act—direct reimbursement for nurse
       practitioners and clinical nurse specialists under Medicare.
       Omnibus Budget Reconciliation Act.
       New provisions under the Rural Health Clinic Services Act.
       Establishment of the Agency for Health Care Policy and Research
       (AHCPR) under the Public Health Service.
       Medicare coverage for screening Pap smears.

1990   Medigap Law to regulate sale of Medicare supplemental policies (so-
       called Medigap policies).
       Americans with Disabilities Act.
       Comprehensive AIDS Resources Emergency Act.
       Medicare Organ Procurement Act.
       Vaccine and Immunizations Amendments.
       TB Prevention Act.
       Drug Treatment Rehabilitation Act.
       National Health Services Revitalization Act.
       Trauma Care Systems and Development Act.
       Homeless Assistance Amendments Act for health services for
       homeless.
       Transition Housing for Substance Abusing Veterans Act.
       Authorization for research on DES.

Table 3.5 (Continued)

Omnibus Budget Reconciliation Act of 1990.

Medicaid eligibility expansions.

Medicaid continuation for women and infants.

Safe Medical Devices Act requires medical device user facilities to report medical device-related deaths, serious illness and injuries.

1991   Patient Self-Determination Act—health care providers must supply all adult patients with written information about their rights and document any advanced directives.

Bill for homeless persons with AIDS.

Women's Health Equity Act introduced.

1992   The Pacific Yew Act to assure a supply of Taxol, drug used in treating ovarian and breast cancer.

Acts to regulate mammography equipment.

Act for goal setting for Native Americans.

Reorganization Act for ADAMHA.

Reauthorization of Older Americans Act.

Revision of Medicaid Discount Drug Law.

Preventive Health Amendments Block Grants for states tied to Healthy People 2000 goals.

Act that renamed CDC.

1993   Family and Medical Leave Act.

---

* Sources for this table include *American Journal of Nursing (1982-93); The American Nurse (1983-1993); The Nation's Health (1983-1993); American Journal of Public Health (1984-1993); Capital Update (1987-1993), Journal of the American Academy of Nurse Practitioners, 1990; Community Health Nursing Council Communique,* American Nurses Association, 1989; *Health Legislation and Regulation,* 1988-1991.

---

renewal. Although some funds continued to trickle down from the federal level, many of the original clinics had to be closed for lack of funds (1, pp. 50-51).

The next major piece of health legislation was the Social Security Act of 1935. Drafted under the Committee on Economic Security, it was a response to pressing social needs prompted by the Depression. Under that act, provisions were made for old age and survivors' assistance, child health care, aid to crippled children, and some general public health measures. Clauses that would have established a plan for national health insurance were defeated. The act did manage to contain provision for federal aid to states for support of dependent children and provision of medical care to women and their newborn infants (1, p. 68).

The Hill-Burton Act of 1946, the Hospital Survey and Construction Act, Public Law 79-725, was designed to improve population-bed ratios, especially in rural areas, as well as to provide for upgrading existing facilities and standards. Monies were made available for state surveys, for planning, and for matching grants for constructing and equipping public and voluntary health institutions. Amendments between 1949 and 1970 provided additional funds and programs and included monies for research and demonstration projects by the Public Health Service. In 1964, the Hospital and Medical Facilities Amendments added grants for more construction and renovation and for neighborhood health centers and emergency room facilities (17, pp. 353-355).

In 1946, the National Mental Health Act was passed and the National Institute of Mental Health was established. Amendments to the Social Security Act, passed in 1950, allowed for payments to vendors (agencies or providers) for medical services and for old age assistance payments to persons in public medical institutions (18, pp. 96, 98).

In 1960, the Kerr-Mills bill was passed. This provided federal aid to states to cover part of the costs of medical services to the indigent aged (19, p. 32). In 1963, the Health Professions Assistance Act provided monies for students in health professions for education.

The Economic Opportunity Act of 1964 created the Office of Economic Opportunity (OEO), which in turn funded neighborhood health centers (12, pp. 222-223).

The Nurse Training Act, Public Law 88-581, of that same year provided direct support for students and schools, funds for constructing facilities, and support for demonstration projects (20, pp. 104-105).

The 89th Congress has been referred to as the health congress. During that session, no fewer than 15 laws affecting health were passed. The most notable of these was Medicare, Public Law 89-97, Title 18 of the Social Security Act, providing medical health insurance for citizens age 65 and over, to be administered through the Social Security Administration (21, p. 161). Medicaid, Title 19 of the Social Security Act, Public Law 89-97, was passed in 1965 as well, providing for a program of medical assistance for the indigent, financed by state and federal funds, and implemented at the state level. In essence, this bill provides for 50 different medical assistance programs, since each state may determine eligibility and, within federal mandates, which services will be offered.

Nineteen sixty-five was also the year of Public Law 89-239, establishing Regional Medical Programs. Monies under this program were directed toward regional cooperation, most of the grantees being universities.

Other significant health-related legislation passed in 1965 is included in Table 3.5.

The Public Health Service Act amendments of 1966 and 1967, Public Laws 89-749 and 90-174, provided monies for planning for health care, with project grants to states (17, pp. 359-360).

The Health Manpower Act of 1968 provided more monies for schools of nursing, and the Nurse Training Act of 1971 authorized capitation grants to nursing schools to increase enrollment and also supported advanced education for certain nurses and nurse practitioners (20, p. 105).

The 1972 amendments to the Social Security Act further defined benefits under Medicare and Medicaid and established the Professional Standards Review Organization (PSRO) process for physicians.

In 1973, the HMO (Health Maintenance Organization) Act, Public Law 92-222, was an attempt to provide a model for prepaid health care agencies. Funds for demonstration projects are included in the act. Subsidies are provided to develop health services for the poor and for rural citizens (22, p. 2).

Thus, federal involvement has escalated in recent years, for between 1961 and 1968, Congress passed 138 laws and appropriation bills dealing with health matters (1, p. 58).

The most monumental piece of federal health legislation of the decade of the 1970s was the National Health Planning and Resources Development Act of 1974, Public Law 93-641. Administered by the Bureau of Health Planning and Resources Development in the Health Resources Administration of Health, Education, and Welfare, this bill added two titles to the Public Health Service Act. Title 15 established a program for health planning and resources development and Title 16 revised the existing Hill-Burton program and authorized funds for development of health resources (23, p. 1). It expanded and replaced three previous bills — Hill-Burton of 1946, Regional Medical Program of 1965, and Comprehensive Health Planning Program of 1966.

The act established a 15-member advisory council on health, education, and welfare to advise, consult with, and make recommendations to the Secretary of Health, Education, and Welfare on health planning.

The act provides for establishing Health Systems Agencies (HSAs) to be responsible for health planning and development within designated areas. These may be private, nonprofit corporations, public regional planning bodies, or units of local government. Whatever the structure, their intent is to improve all aspects of health care delivery, prevent duplication of services, and restrain cost escalation. They are to be governed by a body of no fewer than 10 and no more than 30 members, of whom 60 percent must be resident consumers of the area.

The governor of each state was to designate health service areas — geographic regions appropriate for planning and having a population of 500,000 to 3 million. There was then to be a Health Systems Agency for each health service area. By 1979, a network of 205 health services areas had been designated by state governors and approved by Health, Education, and Welfare (24, p. 2). The governor was also to designate a state Health Planning and Development Agency for health planning and to coordinate efforts of the Health Systems Agencies. Monies were allocated in the bill for health facility construction and renovation (23). HSAs have emerged as major planning units for long-term care.

This bill has profound implications for nursing. One must ask such questions as: How many nurses will be needed and will there be enough? What roles will nurses play? What will be the functions of professional nurses? How many will be needed who have had additional preparation as teachers, administrators, researchers, and planners? In what settings will nurses be found? What sort of reimbursement schemes for nursing will evolve? Where will nurses fit into health teams? Nurses need to be involved as members of Health Systems Agency boards and subarea councils, and as staff in Health Systems Agencies and state health coordinating councils. Nurses also need to work through their state professional organizations in influencing the Health Services Plan for their Health Systems Agencies (26).

In 1976, the National Health Consumer and Health Promotion Act was passed and the Office of Health Information was established.

In late 1977, the Rural Health Clinic Services Act, Public Law 95-210, was passed. This bill provides financial support for health service facilities in rural areas utilizing primary care providers other than physicians and authorizing Medicaid and Medicare payments for services by physician assistants and nurse practitioners (27, p. 1).

Between 1981 and 1993, several significant pieces of legislation were proposed or passed (see Table 3.5). The most significant was P.L. 98-21, an amendment to the Social Security Act establishing a prospective payment system under Medicare. This system, implemented on October 1, 1983, is based on diagnosis-related groups (DRGs) as a means of categorizing clients according to illnesses (28).

Other major pieces of legislation have been passed in efforts to extend Medicaid benefits to more persons, particularly pregnant women, infants, and children, to provide broader third-party reimbursement through Medicaid and Medicare to health care professionals   besides physicians, and to strengthen patients' rights. In spite of a less than receptive executive branch during the 80's, numerous bills were introduced into Congress in an effort to reform the health care delivery system. None of these succeeded in doing that, and as health costs continued to escalate faster than the inflation rate and the number of uninsured and underinsured Americans increased, health care reform became a major issue for the 1992 presidential campaign. Each of the candidates had a plan for reform that was widely publicized as early as the primaries (53). As we go to press, a task force is working on a health care reform plan that is scheduled to be presented to Congress before the end of 1993. Leaders in nursing are working to assure that the voice of nurses will be heard as the plans for reform are shaped (54).

National Health Insurance/National Health Service

Plans for national health insurance are not the creation of contemporary administrations and politicians. Public discussion of a plan for national health insurance can be traced to around 1912 when President Theodore Roosevelt's Progressive Party included such a plan as a plank of the party's platform. Congress even held hearings in 1916 on a plan to include benefits for sickness and for invalids (21, pp. 179-180). From 1915 to 1920 the American Medical Association was considering a plan for compulsory national health insurance and was working on model state plans. During approximately the same period, the American Association for Labor Legislation was attempting to have its model medical care insurance bill passed by legislatures in several states. The opposition of Samuel Gompers, President of the American Federation of Labor, to such a plan did little to expedite its adoption (30, pp. 293-294). At the 1920 American Medical Association National Convention, delegates unanimously passed a resolution declaring opposition to a national plan of compulsory health insurance (1, p. 63).

A child of the Great Depression, Roosevelt's New Deal included a plan for National Health Insurance within its Keystone Social Security Bill. When it appeared that inclusion of a national health insurance plan might jeopardize passage of the Social Security Bill, it was deleted and the bill passed without it (30, pp. 294-295). In 1939, Senator Robert Wagner of New York introduced a bill which included provisions for constructing health care institutions, giving health care assistance to the poor, and allocating federal subsidies to states with comprehensive health insurance programs. The bill died in committee (31, p. 437). In 1943, the Wagner-Murray-Dingell Bill, which included compulsory federal health insurance, was proposed. In 1948, it was proposed again, backed by then President Truman (32, p. 178). Finally, in 1951, the administration withdrew support for national health insurance and the drive for it waned. Between that time and the passing of Medicaid and Medicare in 1965, the Social Security Act was amended to provide payments to providers for care of those on public assistance. The Kerr-Mills bill of 1960 was a compromise in the long debate.

Health insurance for the aged figured in both the 1960 and 1964 campaigns. In 1968, the American Medical Association sponsored its version of a national health insurance — Medi-credit. In 1970, Senator Edward Kennedy introduced his Health Security Program, with AFL-CIO support (21, p. 181). Since that time, numerous bills and plans have been introduced. The major ones are summarized in Table 3.6.

Proposals during the Carter administration included the Kennedy-Waxman Labor Coalition Scheme, to cover everyone and utilize private insurance carriers, the Long Catastrophic Bill, and the Carter Administration's own proposals. All of these are included in Table 3.6. Since then, many more proposals have been introduced in Congress, as shown on Table 3.6.

Several proposals for a national health service have been suggested over the years by groups including the Medical Committee for Human Rights and the Committee for a National Health Service. David Rutstein proposed a national health service based on the United Kingdom's model as a solution for our present health care woes (33, p. 242-253).

There are those who have argued that health insurance schemes are antiquated and that only a national health service can make health care available for all (34). The predominant proposals at present, however, seem to favor a scheme of health insurance rather than nationalizing the health care delivery system. It remains to be seen whether the President's task force can come up with a plan for health coverage for all Americans.

Considerations in Reviewing Health Reform Proposals

When appraising proposals for health care reform, it is important to utilize definite criteria. These criteria will also help you to articulate clearly to your senators and representative your support for a particular bill. The following list of questions will help you formulate criteria for analyzing bills on national health insurance. Using these questions,* you could even come up with your own bill and use it to judge the others.

1. Benefits. What will be covered—mental and physical health? Will there be time limits, e.g., 180 days in hospital?
2. Coverage. Who will be covered? How soon? For how long (if patient is unemployed or disabled)?
3. How many plans does the scheme involve—one for employees, one for the poor/elderly/uninsured? How about retirees?
4. Who will pay? The client? If so, how and how much? Will there be premiums for the insurance? Will there be deductibles? Will a fee for service be set? How about co-insurance? Will monies come from federal revenues and taxes? From employers? From employees?
5. How will reimbursement for providers be handled? How is quality improvement built into the plan? Who determines rates for reimbursement?
6. Who will administer the program? Private insurance companies? The Department of Health and Human Services? The Social Security Administration? A new structure? A combination of groups for different plans within the scheme?
7. Will it be illness or health insurance? Will the scheme make it beneficial and cost effective to keep people well? How much will be spent on prevention and health programs? Will people have to be sick to be covered?
8. Will the scheme reduce barriers? Increase access? Affect distribution of providers and services?
9. Will the scheme alter present modes of health care delivery? Will it be innovative, efficient, and cost effective?
10. What is the role of the consumer in formulating policy? In administering the plan?
11. Will providers be included in policy making? In quality improvement? Are there provisions to stimulate innovative, humanitarian, and creative care giving? Will there be incentives for continuing education of providers?
12. Are there provisions to control costs without sacrificing quality?
13. How is long-term care covered? Catastrophic illness?

---

* Adapted from Kuzay and Wilson (39), Jonas (31), and Widavsky (41).

Nursing Issues in Health Reform

The American Nurses Association has been deeply concerned with proposals for national health insurance and for health care reform. The president of the ANA, and others, have testified before various subcommittees considering such bills. Barbara Nichols, ANA's president in 1980, in testifying urged inclusion of nursing services in all settings in the Kennedy-Waxman bill. She also pointed out the need for giving priority to maternal and child services (42). National League for Nursing representatives also testified, urging attention to the critical shortage of nurses at that time and the impact it would have on any plan of national health insurance (43). Testimony by Ms. Nichols and others urged that nursing care costs be included as covered benefits, that nurses be included as health educators, that the impact of care by nurse practitioners and nurse midwives on neonatal mortality rates be considered, and that support be given to home health care services (44). The National League for Nursing also issued a policy statement endorsing the eventual establishment of a comprehensive national health insurance program (45). In 1974, the American Nurses Association House of delegates passed a series of 11 resolutions on national health insurance (46).

Ingeborg G. Mauksch, a nurse, represented nursing on the Advisory Committee on National Health Insurance to the then Health, Education, and Welfare Secretary Joseph A. Califano, Jr. That committee developed four plans which were submitted to President Carter in 1978. These plans are summarized in Ms. Mauksch's article on the committee (47). The Carter administration's proposal was derived from the report of this committee.

During the 1980s, numerous pieces of legislation were introduced that would provide schemes for health insurance coverage broader in nature than those presently in place (48).

In 1991, *Nursing's Agenda for Health Care Reform* was developed under the aegis of the American Nurses Association and endorsed by more than 60 nursing and other health care organizations (55, 62). The impetus came three years earlier when the Board of Directors of the American Nurses Association created a task force to develop a policy platform. This task force had representatives from constituent organizations of the ANA, the

Table 3.6 Proposals for National Health Insurance

Name of Bill	Known as	Financing	Benefits	Patient Pays
Health Security Act H.R. 21; S. 3 (AFL-CIO support).	Kennedy-Corman	Half from federal general revenues half from special taxes; 1% of payroll from employees, 2.5% from employers and self-employed.	Institutional services: hospital care, skilled nursing facilities up to 120 days. Diagnosis and treatment: physicians' services, laboratory and x-ray, home health services, prescription drugs (for chronic illnesses), medical appliances and ambulance services. Other services: physical checkups, well-child care, maternity, family planning, dental care (up to age 25), vision care and eyeglasses, hearing care and hearing aids.	None.
Comprehensive Health Insurance Act of 1974 H.R. 4747.	CHIP Rep. Carter	Employer-employee premium payments, with employer paying 75% (65% in first three years); special provisions for small employers and those with high increases in payroll costs.	Institutional services: hospital care, skilled nursing facilities up to 100 days. Diagnosis and treatment: physicians' services, laboratory and x-ray, home health services (up to 100 visits), prescription drugs, medical supplies and appliances. Other services: well-child care, maternity, family planning, dental care (under age 13), hearing care and hearing aids (under age 13).	Annual deductible of $150 per person; 25% coinsurance with annual ceiling of $1,500 per family.
National Health Care Services Reorganization and Financing Act H.R. 1 (AHA support).	Ullman	Employer-employee premium-payments with employer paying at least 75%, federal subsidy for low-income workers and certain small	Institutional services: hospital care up to 90 days, skilled nursing facilities (30 days), health-related custodial nursing home care (90 days). Diagnosis and treatment: physicians' services up to 10 visits, laboratory and x-ray, home health services (100 days), prescription drugs limited to specified conditions, medical	Coinsurance (20 percent) or copayments (up to $5) on most items; special "catastrophic" pro-

Table 3.6 (continued)

Name of Bill	Known as	Financing	Benefits	Patient Pays
		employers; patients enrolling in a health care corporation get 10% subsidy; individuals pay own premium.	supplies and appliances. Other services: physical checkups, well-child care, maternity, dental care (under age 13), vision care and eyeglasses (under age 13).	visions become effective when patient's out-of-pocket expenses reach a specified amount.
Comprehensive Health Care Insurance Act of 1975. H.R. 6222 (AMA supported).	Fulton	Employer-employee premium payments, with employer paying at least 65% of cost; small employers get federal help as do all employers with unusual payroll cost increases; self-employed pay own premiums but are assisted by income-tax credits computed on a sliding scale (the lower the income, the higher the credits). Premiums for unemployed paid for by federal government.	Institutional services: hospital care, skilled nursing facilities to 100 days. Diagnosis and treatment: physicians' services, laboratory and x-ray, home health services, medical supplies and equipment. Preventive and special services: physical checkups, well-child care, maternity, family planning, dental care (under age 18).	Coinsurance of 20% with an annual maximum of $1,500 per individual and $2,000 per family.

		Financing	Services	Deductibles/Coinsurance
National Health Care Act of 1976. H.R. 5990; S. 1438.	Burleson-McIntyre	Employer-employee premium payments, the ratios to be negotiated; low-income workers pay less; self-employed pay entire premium; all participants eligible for special tax deductions.	Institutional services: hospital care, skilled nursing facilities to 180 days. Diagnosis and treatment: physicians' services, laboratory and x-ray, home health care (270 days), prescription drugs, medical supplies and appliances. Other services: well-child care, maternity, family planning, dental care (under age 13, one visit), vision care (under age 13, one visit).	Annual deductible of $100 per person; 20 percent coinsurance on all items, with annual family limit of $1,000.
Catastrophic Health Insurance and Medical Assistance Reform H.R. 10028; S. 2470	Long-Ribicoff	Employers pay 1% payroll tax. Similar provisions for self-employed.	Institutional services: after 60 days, hospital care, skilled nursing facilities up to 100 days. Diagnosis and treatment: after an expenditure of $2,000, physicians' services, lab and x-ray, home and health services, medical supplies and appliances. Other services: none.	First 60 days of hospitalization not covered; first $2,000 in family medical expenses not covered.
National Health Insurance Standards Program Family Health Insurance Plan (Developed by the Nixon Administration). S. 1623; H.R. 7741	Bennett Bill and Byrnes Bill	Employers and employees will share premium costs, with employers eventually paying 75%. Group-rate pools will be set up for state and local government employees, self-employed, small employers and people outside of labor force. For the poor, the plan	Comprehensive coverage including hospital, surgical, extended care, diagnostic work-ups, general and special physician services, maternity and well-child care, health maintenance services, low income family counseling, vision care for children, acute hospital psychiatric services.	Patient pays first $100 of expenses and cost of first two days of hospital care, plus 25% co-payment on first $5,000 of expense. The $100 deductible is eliminated for well baby care and child

Table 3.6 (Continued)

Name of Bill	Known as	Financing	Benefits	Patient Pays
		would pay all costs. A sliding scale of subsidies would apply to families with incomes of $3,000 to $5,000. Social Security and Railroad Retirement recipients will be financed through Social Security taxes and Railroad Retirement contributions.		vision care. Deductibles as well as co-payments are eliminated for the poor and scaled down for near poor. Part B Medicare monthly premium costs are eliminated.
National Health Insurance and Health Services Improvement Program S. 836	Javits Bill	General revenues and new Social Security taxes, shared in 3 equal parts by employers, employees, and the federal gov't. Individuals and employer-employee groups can establish alternative private plans, with financing by employers and employees on a 75%-25% basis.	Comprehensive medical coverage, including hospital stays, extended care, surgical, diagnostic workups, general and special physician services, annual physical examinations, maternity, long term prescription drugs for chronic conditions, dental care for young children, psychiatric care in and out of hospital, medical appliances.	Patient pays first $52 of hospital stay and some copayments for long term hospitalization and convalescent care. For other services patient pays first $50 plus 20% of the bill. Drug copayments are limited to $1 per prescription.

Act	Bill	Financing	Benefits	Cost Sharing
Griffiths AFL-CIO Plan of 1970. H.R. 22.	Griffiths AFL-CIO	Tax on payroll and non-earned income, general federal revenues.	Limitations on most types of benefits. Comprehensive health benefits.	Copayment up to annual maximum of $50 a person; $100 a family.
National Voluntary Medical and Hospital Services Insurance.	Ketchum-Lagomarsino Bill	Flat premium $180/year adults; $90/child; low income 1.8% of income for each adult. Matching federal revenues.	Full coverage – physical, dental, surgery, podiatric surgery, laboratory services, hospital services.	Premiums.
National Health Insurance Act. H.R. 94	Dingell Bill	Proportional income tax.	Physician, dental, podiatric, home nursing, hospital and auxiliary, laboratory services.	Federal reimbursement for "reasonable costs."
National Family Health Protection Act. H.R. 3672	Lujan Bill	5% federal income tax surcharge.	Hospital, extended care, home health, physician services.	No deductibles; no coinsurance; vouchers for all families.
Pettengill Proposal 1969.	Pettengill	Federal and state funds.	Supplement Medicare; replace Medicaid for poor, near poor and high insurance risk.	No premium, no cost.
National Health Standards Act. S. 2644.	Fannin Bill	Employers 50%. Employees contribute; federal gov't.	In-patient hospital, physician, x-ray and laboratory, out-patient drugs, PT, medical devices, ambulance.	Premium in employment.
Comprehensive National Health Care Act of 1975. H.R. 8887.	Young Bill	Social Security taxes.	Skilled nursing facilities, hospital, home health, x-ray and laboratory, routine dental, preventative services, prescription drugs, surgery by specialist.	Social Security tax.
Med. Expense Tax Credit Act. S.600	Brock Bill	Allows tax credits, no financing.	Tax credit for expenses over 15% modified adjusted gross income.	Pays for expenses; deducts tax credit.

Table 3.6 (continued) *

Name of Bill	Known as	Financing	Benefits	Patient Pays
	Kennedy/ Waxman Labor Coalition	Private insurers, HMO's, employers, employees, elderly and poor, Medicare, paid by national insurance plan	Hospital, physician, laboratory and x-ray, ambulance, medical equipment, home health, inpatient psychiatric, outpatient physical and speech services	Premiums through employment
	Long Catastrophic plan	Employer tax, federal tax on cigarettes	For catastrophic illness, after set expenditures out of pocket	Costs until coverage in effect
	Carter Administration	Employer/ employee	Hospital, physician, x-ray and laboratory, poor, aged, disabled covered under new Medicare/Medicaid	Premiums
Mitchell-Kennedy Bill/S.1227	Health American pay or play 2 tier	Premiums cost sharing, federal, state revenues	Unlimited in- and outpatient hospital and physician, prenatal care. Limited preventive and mental health.	Premiums.
Rostenkowski HR 3205	Rostenkowski pay or play 2 tier	Premiums, tax increases, state revenues	Parts A and B of Medicare, pregnancy related services and postnatal care.	Premiums.
Kerrey S 1446	Kerrey single payer 1 tier	Cost sharing, tax increases state revenues	Inpatient and outpatient hospital and physician services, screening tests, Rx drugs, long-term care, limited mental health.	

Russo HR 1300	Universal Health Care Act single payer	Tax increases state revenue long-term care premium	Inpatient hospital, physician, nursing facility, preventive care, Rx drugs, limited mental health.	Premium for long term.
Bentson S1872	Bentson insurance reform multitiered	tax expenditures	Inpatient, outpatient hospital, physician, some preventive.	Premiums.
Chaffee S.1936	Chaffee tax, insurance, malpractice reform multitiered	fed and state revenues	Benefits under future national model plan.	Premiums.
Stark HR 650	Stark Mediplan Health Care Act	2% tax on gross income, employees employers	Medical to cover all Americans.	Premiums.
HR 651	Mediplan long-term act	2% tax on gross income	Long term care for all.	

*These are among dozens of proposals that have been created in the past 12 years.

*Synthesized from Schorr (35, pp. 174-180), Rowland (36), Hall (37, pp. 167-208), Kennedy (38, pp. 234- 251), Krizay and Wilson (39, pp. 157-160), and *Legislative Roundup* (40, pp. 1-12): *The American Nurse*, 1992; *Capital Update*, 1991; *Journal of the American Academy of Nurse Practitioners*, 1991; *The Nation's Health*, 1991-1992.

Table 3.7. Key Features of Nursing's Agenda for Health Care Reform*

Access for all citizens and residents	Citizens, lawful residents, aliens.
Access to alternative providers	Nurses, nurse practitioners, clinical nurse specialists, nurse-midwives, etc.
Federally mandated set of basic services	Primary health care, hospital care. Emergency care, inpatient and outpatient professional, home care services. Prevention services, speech, hearing, dental and eye care up to age 18. Prescription drugs, medical supplies and equipment, lab and radiologic services. Mental health, substance abuse rehab. Hospice care. Long-term care services of relatively short duration. Restorative services.
Emphasize health promotion/prevention	Prenatal, perinatal, well child care. School-based disease prevention. Health screening.
Catastrophic coverage for long-term care	Limits on out-of-pocket individual costs.
Special programs for disadvantaged	Healthstart (like Head Start) for special groups such as low-birthweight babies, battered and neglected kids, kids exposed to violence, homelessness. Expanded WIC program, programs for infants and children, other special programs for the most vulnerable.
Initial emphasis on women and kids under 6	Pregnant women; infants and children.
Co-payment, deductibles retained.	Reduce or eliminate for low income families.
Employer mandated coverage; everyone must be covered by one of these options	Public plan administered by states for the poor (those below 200% federal poverty level); individuals and employers can opt for this. Private plans—employment based health benefit plans and commercial health insurance.

Table 3.7   (Continued)

Subsidized rate for employers with <25 employees	Can buy into public plan.
Combine public programs into single plan	One public plan accessible as above.
Encourage managed care and case management	Organized delivery systems to link financing of care to delivery of services. Public plan—must enroll in approved provider networks. Variety of providers to act as case managers to integrate, coordinate, and advocate for persons needing extensive services.
Covers long-term care of short duration	Variety of public and private options to prevent impoverishing patients and their families.
Health care delivery in community	Whenever possible in familiar settings, including schools, homes, places of work, other community locales.
Insurance reforms including community ratings	Community ratings for all insurers. Cap on out-of-pocket for catastrophic; reinsurance pools to protect state insurers and consumers against high costs.
Administrative reforms to reduce costs	Outcome and effectiveness measures to reduce litigation and reduce defensive practices.
Practice and outcome guidelines	Derived from research, carefully weigh costs, benefits of new innovative approaches; use advancements in clinical practice and technology.
States maintain health care funding levels	States have authority to modify implementation to reflect geographic diversity.
Identifies costs and sources of revenue	Costs included in proposal; dividends to be reaped over time with more emphasis on prevention. Individuals, employers and government will share funding.

* Synthesized from *Nursing's Agenda for Health Care Reform,* American Nurses Association, 1991; *Capital Update,* 1991, 9, p. 4; E. Reifsnider, Restructuring the American health care system: An analysis of Nursing's Agenda for Health Care Reform, *Nurse Practitioner,* 1992, 17(5):65,69-70,72,75.

American Academy of Nursing, and other nurses, including representatives from nurses in the government. In 1989, the National League of Nursing's national health proposal had been drafted (58), and in early 1990, the Tri Council (consisting of the ANA, the American Organization of Nurse Executives, and the American Association of Colleges of Nursing) came up with a plan to join forces to draft a plan. As the plan began to take shape, the constituent organizations of the ANA and the National Organization Liaison Forum (NOLF) gave input, and the document then went to the Tri Council (55, 56, 57). The major premises of nursing's agenda appear in Table 3.7.

Physicians have begun to consider plans for health care reform, and the two major physician groups, the American Medical Association and the American College of Physicians, have made public their proposals (59). In addition to members of Congress and professional organizations, major providers of health care have also created proposals for reform (60). One of these is a major HMO, Harvard Community Health Plan (61).

It has become increasingly clear to providers and consumers of health care that a balanced budget for the nation is tied to health care reform. In the chapter on paying for care, this will become obvious. Whatever the outcome of the current task force on health care reform, the 1990s is sure to be a landmark decade for health care in the United States and for health care legislation at the federal level.

While it is not clear whether we will have a national plan by the end of this century, what is clear is that nurses and nursing will play a significant role in whatever plan might evolve (49). "Nurses know that U.S. citizens can get better access to better health care at affordable costs" (50). And nurses are becoming increasingly vocal about health care policy, about how a future health care system might look, and their roles in that system (50).

Summary

It should be apparent from the foregoing pages that health legislation at the federal level, as well as at the state and local levels, can influence the course of delivery of services for clients and providers. It is, therefore, incumbent on us as providers and consumers to influence the direction health legislation may take. As nurses we have to collectively lobby, vote, and in every possible and legal way let our views be know. Only then will we have earned our right to a position as major creators of health policies.

References

1. Cray, E. (1970). In Failing Health. Indianapolis: Bobbs-Merrill
2. Bagwell, M. and Clements, S. (1985). A Political Handbook for Health Professionals. Boston: Little, Brown.
3. Donley, Sr. R. (1979). An inside view of the Washington health scene. American Journal of Nursing 79(11):1946-1949.
4. Billings, G. (1975). American Nurses Association in the nation's capital. American Journal of Nursing 75(7):1182-1183.
5. Feldstein, P.J. (1977). Health Associations and the Demand for Legislation: The Political Economy of Health. Cambridge, MA: Ballinger.
6. N-CAP. (1980). Nurses, Register and Vote for a Healthy U.S.A.! Washington, DC: N-CAP.
7. Ellis, J.R. and Hartley, C.L. (1992). Nursing in Today's World. 4th ed. Philadelphia: Lippincott.
8. Burke, S. (1979). What the Washington professionals expect. American Journal of Nursing 79(11):1949.
9. Stimpson, M. and Hanley, B. (1991). Nurse policy analyst. Nursing & Health Care 12(1):10-15.
10. Sharp, N., Biggs, S., and Wakefield, M. (1991). New opportunities for nurses. Nursing & Health Care 12(1):16-22.
11. Wilmer, D.M., Walkley, R.P., and O'Neill, E.J. (1978). Introduction to Public Health. New York: Macmillan.
12. Wigley, R. and Cook, J.R. (1975). Community Health Concepts and Issues. New York: Van Nostrand.
13. Dock, L.L. and Stewart, I.M. (1938). A Short History of Nursing. 4th ed. New York: Putnam's Sons.
14. Freymann, J.G. (1974). The American Health Care System: Its Genesis and Trajectory. New York: MEDCOM Press.
15. Forgotson, E.H. (1967). 1965: The turning point in health law—1966 reflections. American Journal of Public Health 57:934-935.
16. Maternal and Child Health Service-HEW-PHS (1971). First Federal Law Passed Against Lead Poisoning. Rockville, MD: U.S. Department of Health, Education, and Welfare, Public Health Service, Health Services and Mental Health Administration, Maternal and Child Health Service.
17. McCarthy, C. (1977). Planning for health care. In: S. Jonas, ed., Health Care Delivery in the United States. New York: Springer.
18. Thomas, W.C. (1969). Nursing Homes and Public Policy. Ithaca, NY: Cornell University Press.

19. Law, S.A. (1964). Blue Cross: What Went Wrong? New Haven: Yale University Press.
20. Barhydt, N.R. (1977). Nursing. In: S. Jonas, ed., Health Care Delivery in the United States. New York: Springer.
21. Somers, A.R. and Somers, H.M. (1977). Health and Health Care Policies in Perspective. Germantown, MD: Aspen Systems.
22. National League for Nursing. (1978). Health Maintenance Organizations. Public Affairs Advisory. New York: National League for Nursing.
23. HEW-PHS. (1976). Health Planning and Resources Development Act of 1974. Hyattsville, MD: U.S. Department of Health, Education, and Welfare, Public Health Service, Health Resources Administration.
24. National League for Nursing. (1979). Update from Capitol Hill. Public Affairs Advisory. New York: National League for Nursing.
25. Novello, D.J. (1976). The National Health Planning and Resources Development Act. Nursing Outlook 24(6):354-358.
26. Chopoorian, T. and Craig, M.M. (1976). Public Law 93-641: Nursing and health care delivery. American Journal of Nursing 76(12):1988-1991.
27. HEW. (1979). Rural Health Clinic Services. Washington, DC: U.S. Department of Health, Education, and Welfare.
28. American Journal of Nursing. (1983). HHS is set to go with prospective payment proposal for Medicare. American Journal of Nursing 83(2):195, 208, 210, 212.
29. American Journal of Nursing. (1983). Prospective reimbursement to be in effect this year for Medicare. American Journal of Nursing 83(5):697, 710.
30. Marmor, T.R. (1976). Origins of the government health insurance issues. In: D. Kotelchuck, ed., Prognosis Negative. New York: Vintage Books, pp. 293-303.
31. Jonas, S. (1977). National health insurance. In: S. Jonas, ed., Health Care Delivery in the United States. New York: Springer, pp.436-466.
32. Ehrenreich, B. and Ehrenreich, J. (1970). The American Health Empire: Power, Profits, and Politics. New York: Vintage Books.
33. Rutstein, D.D. (1974). Blueprint for Medical Care. Cambridge, MA: MIT Press.
34. Terris, M., Cornely, P.B., Daniels, H.C., and Kerr, L.E. (1977). The case for a national health service. American Journal of Public Health 67(12):1183-1185.
35. Schorr, D. (1970). Don't Get Sick in America. Nashville: Aurora.
36. Rowland, H.S. and Rowland, B.L. (1978). The Nurses Almanac. Germantown, MD: Aspen Systems.
37. Hall, T.D. (1976). Proposals under consideration. In: New Directions in Public Health Care. San Francisco: Institute for Contemporary Studies.
38. Kennedy, E.M. (1972). In Critical Condition. New York: Simon and Schuster.
39. Krizay, J. and Wilson, A. (1974). The Patient as Consumer. Lexington, MA: Lexington Books.
40. American Medical Association. (1976). National Health Insurance.

Legislative Roundup. Chicago: American Medical Association.
41. Wildavsky, A. (1977). Doing better and feeling worse: The political pathology of health policy. Daedalus 106(1):105-124.
42. Bauknecht, V.L. (1980). American Nurses Association testifies on national health insurance. The America Nurse 12(3):2.
43. National League for Nursing. (1980). McNulty addresses nursing shortage in national health insurance testimony. NLN News 28(3):7.
44. Brewer, K. (1979). Inclusion of nursing services vital to any national health insurance plan. The American Nurse ll(1):1-2, 16.
45. National League for Nursing. (1979). NLN Position statement on national health insurance. National League for Nursing, Pub. No. 11-1786.
46. Bowman, R.A. and Culpepper, R.C. (1975). National health insurance: Some of the issues. American Journal of Nursing 75(11):2017-2021.
47. Mauksch, I.G. (1978). On national health insurance. American Journal of Nursing 78(8):1323-1327.
48. The Nation's Health. (1988). Kennedy offers hope for health insurance plan. The Nation's Health 18(12):8.
49. Harrington, C.A. (1988). A national health care program: Has its time come? Nursing Outlook 36:214-216,255.
50. Huey, F.L. (1988). How nurses would change U.S. health care. American Journal of Nursing 88:1482-1493.
51. Cohen, W.J. and Milburn, L.T. (1988). What every nurse should know about political action. Nursing & Health Care 9:294-297.
52. Davis, G.C. (1988). Nursing values and health care policy. Nursing Outlook 36:289-292.
53. Healthcare Tends and Transition. (1992). Proposals from the Presidential candidates. Healthcare Trends and Transition 3(6):20-21.
54. Mikulencak, M. (1993). Staff nurses speak out on reform. The American Nurse 25(3):2.
55. American Nurses Association. (1991). Nursing's Agenda for Health Care Reform. (1991). Washington, DC: American Nurses Association.
56. Reifsnider, E. (1992). Restructuring the American health care system: An analysis of nursing's agenda for health care reform. The Nurse Practitioner 17(5):65,69-70,72,75.
57. Nursing introduces its national health strategy to the public. National League for Nursing Public Policy Bulletin, March, 1991.
58. NLSs National Health Strategy: A Plan for Reform. National League for Nursing Public Policy Bulletin, Fall, 1990.
59. Physicians' group calls for national health care budget. (1992). The Nation's Health 22(10:1,17.
60. Other plans from the public policy and health arenas. (1992). Healthcare Trends and Transition 3(6):23.
61. Who will cure America's health care crisis? Harvard Community Health Plan Annual Report 1991. Brookline, MA: Harvard Community Health Plan.
62. Cassetta, R.A. (1993). Coalitions bring quality to health care reform. The American Nurse 25(1):7.

4

Subsystems in
Health Care Delivery

The U.S. health care delivery system has a number of interesting subsystems, some of which will be examined in this chapter. Their importance to the overall delivery system is significant for a number of reasons.

Some of these subsystems are examples of the federal government's involvement in hands-on care, and they function under Congressional imperatives. Even though this role may be less public than the legislative or payment functions assumed by Washington, it is an important one. Other subsystems are unique in that they differ in structure and function from traditional delivery models, both private and public. The roles nurses play in some of these are different from those in private, voluntary, nonprofit settings.

The examples we have chosen underscore the diversity of our complex health care delivery megasystem. Some also reveal the influences of consumer groups. For example, veterans, persons with AIDS, and persons with disabilities have had an enormous impact on the creation of care delivery systems and how care is delivered.

The Department of Veterans Affairs:
Veterans' Health Services

The Veterans Administration (VA) was founded in 1930 and now serves an estimated 27 million service veterans. One-third of the U.S. population has an immediate family involvement in veterans affairs. Under the law creating the new Department of Veterans Affairs in 1988, the Veterans Health Services and Research Administration was created, subsuming the VA health care system (2).

The health services arm of the VA comprises 172 medical centers, 233 outpatient clinics, 27 domiciliaries for the chronically ill, 194 veteran centers, and is the nation's largest health care system. (1, 2). It is organized into 27 VA medical districts, with long-term units, nursing home facilities, and coordination of other services which may include those for spinal cord injury, neurology, medicine, rehabilitation, radiology, AIDS, and nuclear medicine. Tertiary programs include those for drug dependency, hemodialysis, the homeless, chronically mentally ill, transplants, speech, aphasia, prosthesis, and home care.

Eligibility for veteran's health care benefits is extended to any veteran who incurred a service-connected disability and who received an honorable or general discharge. In 1978, benefits were extended to certain individuals who served in the Merchant Marine during World War II. Admission may be through outpatient clinics, private physician referral, direct application, and humanitarian and congressional intervention.

The organization of care within the VA system is oriented toward self-care. It is not uncommon to see hospitalized clients going to the x-ray department or other treatment area on guerneys or wheelchairs by themselves. They may make their own beds and help each other. Most large VA facilities have a barber shop, canteen, commissary, and other services accessible to clients as well as staff and visitors.

Since its inception, the veterans' health facilities have played an active role in the education of providers, offering clinical experien- ces for medical, nursing, and other students, and participating in intern and residency programs. VA medical facilities provide clinical rotations to one out of three physicians and one out of four professional nurses.

The VA health care system employs more than 37,000 nurses and countless other health care personnel. It is the largest hospital system in the nation and the largest independent federal agency.

Nursing in the VA

Nurses in the VA work under a position grading system. They can attain a higher grade through formal continuing education, work evaluation, years of service, and meeting specified criteria for job performance (3). Pamphlets provided by the VA spell out expectations and benefits for employees (3). Important information is generally communicated in writing, and job descriptions, memos, and the *VA Employee Letter* keep all employees, including nurses, up to date on policies, benefits, requirements, advancement data, and so on. Most if not all of the VA facilities employing nurses have a written philosophy and objectives for nursing service, a written chain of command, and important policies which are shared with prospective employees. Nursing service within the VA system is comprised of research, education, and service. There are opportunities for clinical practice, administration, research, and education in VA nursing positions (3).

The Military

The federal government assumes responsibility for the health care of all military personnel on active duty and their dependents and survivors, and for retirees and their dependents and survivors. Military facilities range from medical stations and field hospitals to large general facilities such as Walter Reed Hospital and Bethesda Naval Hospital.

The health services for the military are administered by the Department of Defense. The Navy has many stateside hospitals and medical centers, as well as over a dozen in U.S. territories and overseas. It also maintains numerous branch clinics and dispensaries, as well as health facilities aboard ships. The Army has more than 40 hospitals and medical centers, as well as countless smaller facilities in foreign countries where there are U.S. Army installations (6). The Air Force maintains six medical centers stateside and over 150 small clinics, dispensaries, and aid stations at bases abroad. The military health services collectively represent what is probably the most extensive example of socialized medicine in the U.S.

In addition to the on-base facilities of the three branches of the military, CHAMPUS (Civilian Health and Medical Program for the Uniformed Services) provides financing for medical care for dependents, survivors, and retirees and their dependents, and a small number of selected U.S. Public Health Service employees. These benefits are extended only when base facilities are not available or accessible. CHAMPUS is similar to Medicare in having deductible and coinsurance clauses, although it is more comprehensive in its coverage. It is financed directly through the budget of the Department of Defense. It sets fee profiles in order to avoid unreasonable charges for services by providers (7).

Nursing in the Military

The military health services utilize medical paraprofessional personnel extensively for direct care of clients. The medical technicians ("medics") of the Air Force, and the corpspersons of the Navy and Army are prepared to provide a range of services. They act as nursing and medical assistants in situations when professionals are available. In combat or on a ship within a fleet, these "medics" are often the *only* health care providers.

Such use of nonprofessional personnel constitutes a challenge to nurses responsible for or overseeing the care rendered. The role of military medical corpspersons also contributed to the evolution of the role of physicians's assistant, sometimes confused with that of the nurse practitioner.

Nurses form a vital part of the military and medical services. Women volunteers served as nurses to our military as far back as the American Revolution. These untrained nurses were, indeed, the founders of the nursing services for our military. It is ironic, then, that nurses have gained their rightful place as permanent commissioned officers only recently.

The Army Nurse Corps was founded in 1901 and the Navy Nurse Corps in 1908. The Air Forces Nurse Corps was founded in 1949 as part of the Air Force Medical Service (8, p. 247). When the Army Reorganization Bill establishing the Army Nurse Corps was passed by Congress in 1901, nurses were given letters of appointment and were to agree to serve three years; their rank and functions were not defined, however (9, p. 286). Canadian nurses had possessed officer rank since 1906, so after World War I nurses of the American military decided to press for change. As a result, relative rank was given to nurses (8, p. 291 through a bill passed by Congress in 1920 and signed by President Woodrow Wilson (8, p. 149).

A new branch of military nursing was spawned by World War II. The advent of extensive air warfare and air evacuation of the wounded gave birth to aeromedical nurses or flight nurses (8, p. 155). Another outgrowth of World War II was the granting of commissioned rank in both services; the act granting permanent commissioned rank for Army and Navy nurses was signed in 1947 (8, p. 159). It should be noted that the Chief Nurses of the Air Force and Army now hold the rank of Brigadier General and that the Chief Nurse of the Navy is an Admiral. Although the Nurse Corps lags behind the Medical Corps in number of nurses in upper ranks, progress is being made in that direction.

During World War II there was much discussion about drafting nurses, but no decision was made before the close of the war. With the action in Korea of the early '50s, the House of Delegates of the American Nurses' Association finally gave authorization for its board to support legislation for conscription of nurses in times of national emergency (8, p. 160).

All three Nurse Corps require graduation from a state approved and preferably National League of Nursing accredited school of nursing. The criteria for each service are spelled out in detail. Age requirements vary somewhat, depending upon the service, as do rank, basic training, and type and location of assignment. The Navy enlists new nursing school graduates between the ages of 20 and 35, and the Army and Air Force enlist nurses up to age 35. Nurses with experience who are over the age limit may be accepted with advanced rank commensurate with experience. The Navy requires a baccalaureate degree or a minimum of 12 months nursing experience after graduation. The Army now also requires a baccalaureate degree and the Air Force requires a B.A. or B.S.N. in the sciences. It is possible to enlist in the Army or Air Force Reserves without having served on active duty, after a period of basic training. It is also possible to enlist in ROTC programs prior to graduation. Professional nurse registration in at least one state is required for duty entry. Nurses in the military are required to maintain standards of physical fitness and readiness for defense, and to engage in continuing education programs (10, 11, 12)

Several contributions and challenges to nursing from the military should be noted. The services rewarded experience and education with commensurate and equal rank and pay earlier than did civilian institutions, either medical or educational. Many advances in emergency care and nursing support of disaster victims prior to and during evacuation can be attributed to wartime experiences. Nurses continue to push the frontiers of knowledge development through more recent wartime experiences in the Persian Gulf and Somalia (5).

We can attribute some of our nursing traditions and heritage to military influence. Conversely, nursing has contributed a great deal to the welfare of our armed forces. The value of well-prepared nurses was never more evident to the military than at the close of World War I (9, p. 288). The reputation gained by nurses in World War II assured them a permanent role in our military and paved the way for permanent commissioned status in all the corps. The heritage of the hundreds of nurses decorated for special service following World War II is that upon which modern military nursing is founded. The nursing practice model of the Army Nurse Corps is one that has merit in civilian systems as well (4).

U.S. Public Health Service as Provider

The federal government is also involved as a direct provider of health services through the Public Health Service. The National Institutes of

Health operates a 540-bed clinical center for research. The Centers for Disease Control and Prevention respond to calls for aid from around the country. Under the Health Resources and Services Administration, the National Health Service Corps recruits health professionals and places them in areas of critical need. The Indian Health Service is another example of direct service under Health and Human Services. The Bureau of Health Care Delivery and Assistance serves as the liaison between the Public Health Service and the Federal Bureau of Prisons, the Coast Guard, and other groups for whom the Public Health Service has traditionally provided health services. The Substance Abuse and Mental Health Services Administration, through the National Institute of Mental Health, administers Saint Elizabeth's Hospital in Washington, D.C. (15). Each of these will be described as examples of government involvement in direct provision of hands-on care.

National Health Service Corps

The National Health Service Corps was begun in 1972 to reach out to areas with critical shortages of health personpower. It was revitalized in 1990 with funding allocations and authorization to the year 2000. Corps members represent various professions: nursing, medicine, dentistry, and allied health care disciplines. The corps has provided over 16,000 professionals serving in hundreds of sites in all 10 USPHS regions. Members are assigned to communities where they provide direct care and help the citizens establish a system of health care delivery. As of 1991, 2,082 primary care, 796 dental, and 625 mental health professional shortage areas (HPSAs) had been designated in the U.S.; most of these were designated geographically but also by specific population group and facilities.

The first corps team was a couple, a physician and nurse, assigned to a community in northern Maine. The corps also encourages professionals assigned to underserved areas to set up practice in those areas after completion of their education and/or time with the corps (23). The corps is staffed through scholarships and stipends for professionals who must then agree to give two years of service in an underserved area for each year of scholarship, with a minimum of two years (13). There is also a federal loan repayment program with a two-year commitment.

Indian Health Service

Health services for Native Americans were originally under the aegis of the War Department and then, in 1849, the Department of the Interior. The Bureau of Indian Affairs, established in 1834, was assigned the task of "civilizing" the Indians and, incidentally, with providing them with health care. Health services were fragmented and oriented toward control of prevalent diseases, among them trachoma and tuberculosis, until the responsibility for Indian health was transferred to the Public Health Service in 1955. Since that time, the Indian Health Service, elevated to the status of an agency in the Public Health Service in 1988, has been providing care for more than one million Native Americans and Alaskan Natives. It operates 43 hospitals, 66 large health centers, 60 health stations, and five school health stations, most of which are in rural and remote areas. Tribal groups operate seven hospitals, 73 health centers, and 240 clinics. The evolving model is for tribes to manage their own health care facilities (17).

Since the Public Health Service takeover, health services for native Americans have expanded rapidly, appropriations for health care have risen sharply, life expectancy has increased, and infant mortality has decreased. In spite of this, the effects of poverty, malnutrition, and the hazards of poor housing and unsafe work as still there, as are the feelings of isolation from the mainstream of society (16).

There is a strong commitment within the Indian Health Service to recruit more health care professionals of Indian descent. Although more than half of the employees of that service are now of Indian descent, more Indian professionals are needed. In addition, the Service is committed to improving health and to involving its clients in making decisions concerning their care (14).

More than 2,000 nurses are employed in the Indian Health Service (15). Opportunities are available for nursing students to spend summers working in Indian Health Service facilities. In addition, nurses may apply to these facilities to work one or more years after graduation. (See chapter 7.)

Bureau of Health Care Delivery and Assistance

The Bureau of Health Care Delivery and Assistance operates the Gillis Long Center for Hansen's disease, and is responsible for all medical programs for the Coast Guard and for health care in the federal prison system (15). Nurses employed in these Public Health Service hospitals and clinics are federal employees and receive benefits as such, including retirement.

National Institutes of Health

The National Institutes of Health has 16 research institutes and is headquartered in Bethesda, Maryland. It has a 540-bed research hospital and an ambulatory care research facility. The thousands of clients who are referred to National Institutes of Health every year are selected for admission because they are suffering from diseases under current study by one or more of the institutes. The center is designed with laboratory and clinical facilities on the same floors, so that researchers and clinicians can collaborate closely (13, 25). Nurses are among the many professionals employed at National Institutes of Health, both as clinicians and as researchers, most recently to staff the National Institute for Nursing Research, the newest institute of the NIH.

Centers for Disease Control and Prevention

The Centers for Disease Control and Prevention, until 1970 the Communicable Disease Center, is headquartered in Atlanta, Georgia. Appropriately, it is concerned with controlling and preventing disease. It provides personpower help in times of epidemics through disease control and immunization programs, and is responsible for a program devoted to examining coal miners for early signs of "black lung" disease. It is also responsible for quarantine operations. Nurses are among the professionals employed by the Centers for Disease Control and Prevention (15).

Community Health Centers

Neighborhood or community health centers were not an invention of the 1960s. Their history is long and they have experienced an ebb and flow in popularity in response to crises within the system. In the 1920s, the first two centers which might be termed comprehensive were established in New York City's East Harlem and Yorkville. These were funded by the Red Cross and the Milbank Memorial fund. Based on their success, the city was divided into 30 health districts, each to have a center and, under Mayor Laguardia, 7 health centers were built [18].

Community health centers, utilizing consumer input and a health care team approach, have evolved in urban and rural areas over the past two decades in response to the needs of Americans for whom health care was unavailable or inaccessible. Although staffed for the most part by providers from the local population, these facilities are, or were initially, funded by one or more federal agencies or programs. It should be noted that such centers might have one or more professional providers assigned to them from the National Health Service Corps. These centers may be of several types. One is the neighborhood health center, designed to meet the needs of a particular target community in which it is located. Under the federal Office of Economic Opportunity, part of the Johnson era "War on Poverty" from 1964 to 1968, numerous neighborhood health centers were begun (19).

Some of these neighborhood health centers are worth citing as examples. One of the earliest was opened in 1965 at Columbia Point, a high-rise housing project in the Dorchester section of Boston, isolated by a major highway on a desolate point of land jutting out into the bay. This project, initially underwritten by Office of Economic Opportunity funds, was sponsored by Tufts University School of Medicine (20, pp. 178-180). This project developed into a community-oriented, comprehensive health care agency with a great deal of input from the clients it serves (20, pp. 199-200). Most recently, this center merged with another in Boston. The whole project has undergone extensive renovation to make it a more livable and less formidable and isolated place.

Tufts University physicians also founded a rural center in Bolivar County, Mississippi, in 1966. Known as the Mound Bayou project, this center began in a church parsonage. In responding to the intense poverty of the area, the center not only set out to provide health care, but in addition started a farm cooperative and organized crews to attack the most obvious environmental hazards, among them poor sanitation facilities, rats, and an impure water supply (21, pp. 198-199).

The Mile Square Health Center on Chicago's West Side is literally an almost mile-square area that is teeming with poverty and packed with about 25,000 persons, most of whom are Black. This center was established in 1967 under the auspices of St. Luke's Presbyterian Hospital and was reaching over two-thirds of the target population by its third year (21, pp. 137-139).

The center at Montefiore Hospital in the Bronx, New York, was another early project. It is now known as the Martin Luther King Neighborhood Health Center.

By 1970, there were already 49 health centers in this country, extending from New York to California and operating out of a variety of settings ranging from storefronts to sparkling new buildings, one of which arose out of the debris of the 1965 Watts riot (22, p. 144).

An important concept that has been implemented in neighborhood health centers is that of the team approach to health care delivery (19). Nurses, serving in many roles including that of primary care practitioner, are an integral part of these teams.

The Office of Economic Opportunity was disbanded in the 1970s and federal support for the neighborhood centers was subsumed under the Department of Health, Education, and Welfare (now the Department of Health and Human Services). With a concurrent cut in funding, many of these centers have become more dependent upon third-party reimbursement through Medicare, Medicaid, and sliding scale fees (19).

Community health centers continue to exist as subsystems within the cosmos of the United States health care delivery macrosystem. The Bureau of Health Care Delivery and Assistance of the Health Resources and Services Administration, U.S. Public Health Service, continues to support 540 community health centers, serving about 5.1 million persons in communities throughout the country in all territories and states except Wyoming. Approximately half of the clients are in urban areas and half are in rural areas. The National Association of Community Health Centers was founded as a national advocacy organization to assure growth and development of such community-based centers. (15, 24)

For-Profit Subsystems

During the past two decades, several types of for-profit health care delivery systems have evolved. One of these is the freestanding emergi-center or urgent care center, some with names that sound like fast food restaurants. Some of these are truly emergency care centers, open 24 hours a day, seven days a week, and others are open during more conventional business hours, but often include weekends. Known to some as "doc in a box," these centers serve many uninsured persons, those with common short-term illnesses such as ear and urinary tract infections, and fractures. Often care is on a walk-in basis and no appointment is necessary. They are located in shopping centers of town and cities, in shopping malls, and even in transportation centers (19).

Hospitals, birthing centers, nursing homes, long-term care facilities, rehabilitation centers, health maintenance organizations, dialysis centers, breast centers, nutrition centers, ambulatory care centers owned by hospitals or other corporations, home health care services, mental health centers, and the private practices of a variety of health care providers including physicians, nurses, social workers, psychologists, physical therapists, speech therapists, dietitians, occupational therapists, chiropractors, and opticians, all can operate for profit and some of these exist only for profit. These, too, constitute subsystems and figure in the complex megasystem of health care delivery. Most of these are accessible only to persons with health insurance or coverage under one of the federally funded programs, or the ability to pay out-of-pocket.

Summary

The subsystems discussed in this chapter exemplify the diversity and complexity of the U.S. health care macrosystem. Some represent models which have potential for broader application. Others are Band-Aid attempts to cure the ravaging disease plaguing the system as a whole. Some reflect a recycling of earlier attempts at solutions or reform. Each contributes to the total picture of the macrosystem within which nurses function as the largest group of professional care providers. A knowledge and analysis of the component subsystems is part of the database necessary as a precursor to change. Some of these subsystems represent cost effective means of delivering care that are very acceptable to consumers. These may become models for reform.

References

1. Statistical Abstract of the United States. 112th ed. (1992). Washington, DC: U.S. Department of Commerce, Bureau of the Census.
2. VA Today. (1989). Washington, DC: Department of Veterans Affairs.
3. VA Nursing. (1990). Washington, DC: Department of Veterans Affairs.
4. Adams-Ender, C.L., Jennings, B., Bartz, C., and Jensen, R. (1991). Nursing practice models. Nursing and Health Care 12(3):120-123.
5. McGookin, D. (1991). Army nurses—90 years of service. The American Nurse 23(4):15.
6. The Army Health Care Team. (1986). Washington, DC: U.S. Government Printing Office, Pub. 642-361.
7. Krizay, J. and Wilson, A. (1974). The Patient as Consumer: Health Care Financing in the United States. Lexington, MA: Lexington Books, pp. 84-85.
8. Dietz, L.D. (1963). History and Modern Nursing. Philadelphia: F.A. Davis.
9. Dolan, J. (1978). Nursing in Society. 14th ed. Philadelphia: Saunders.

10. Mather, C. (Colonel, U.S. Air Force Reserve Nurse Corps). Personal communication, June, 1980.
11. Hayes, E. (Captain, U.S. Army Reserve Nurse Corps). Personal communication, June, 1980.
12. Navy Nurse Corps. (1981). Washington, DC: Navy Recruiting Command, Recruiting Advertisement Department.
13. The National Health Service Corps serving America's communities. (1992). Summary Fact Sheet.
14. Indian Health Service. (no date). Rockville, MD: U.S. Department of Health and Human Services.
15. U.S. Public Health Service. (no date). McLean, VA: U.S. PHS Recruitment.
16. Indian Health Service. (no date). Rockville, MD: U.S. Department of Health and Human Services, IHS.
17. 1990 budget would maintain services, seeks growth in tribal contracting. (1989). NIHB Health Reporter 4(13):1-3.
18. Alford, R.R. (1975). Health Care Politics. Chicago: University of Chicago Press, pp. 103-104.
19. Jonas, S., Rosenberg, S.N. (1986). Ambulatory care. In: S. Jonas, ed., Health Care Delivery in the United States, 3rd ed. New York: Springer.
20. Bellin, S.S. and Geiger, H.J. (1976). The impact of a neighborhood health center. In: R.L. Kane, J.M. Kasteler, and R.M. Gray, eds., The Health Gap. New York: Springer.
21. Klaw, S. (1975). The Great American Medicine Show. New York: Penguin Books.
22. Schorr, D. (1970). Don't Get Sick in America. Nashville: Aurora.
23. Stamps, P.L. and Kuriger, F.H. (1983). Location decisions of National Health Service Corps physicians. American Journal of Public Health 73(8):906-908.
24. Community Health Centers. (1986). Washington, DC: National Clearinghouse for Primary Care Information.
25. Practice Nursing on the Leading Edge. (1989). Bethesda, MD: National Institutes of Health.

5

Paying for Care

There is an old saying that whoever pays the piper calls the tune. Our health care system is a striking example of the opposite. Although we as tax payers pay a major portion of the health care bill, we often do not call the tune. Incredible as it may seem, expenditures for care often depend on the whims, fancies, or sacred causes of our legislators. It is no accident that priorities have shifted with each election year. Mental health, cancer, arthritis, mental retardation, and so on, all have had their day. In fact, what we have really funded is illness care, but we have continued to refer to "health care" costs in discussions of paying for care (1).

Health Care Costs

Health care expenditures in the United States are roaring toward 14% of the gross national product (GNP), having already surpassed the 12% mark. Health care is now the nation's largest industry.

It has been predicted that by the year 2000, health care costs will consume more than 16% of the gross national product if we continue on our present course (15). In 1930, these costs took only 4% of the GNP (2, p. 12). Figure 5.1 illustrates the changes over the past three

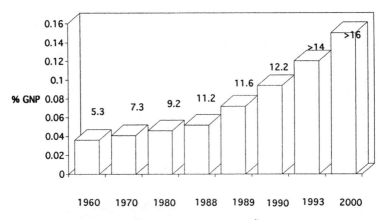

Fig. 5.1. Health care spending as a percent of GNP. *

decades. Left unchecked, the rise in health care costs will continue
to exceed both the general rate of inflation and the rise in consumer
prices (Figure 5.2). Between 1950 and 1976, while consumer prices

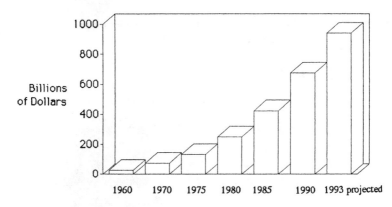

Fig. 5.2. National health spending.

* Except where otherwise noted, tables, figures, and charts in this chapter come from a synthesis
of information from: *The Nation's Health,* 1991 and 1992; The Bureau of Labor Statistics, Health
Care Financing Administration, 1993; General Accounting Office, 1991; *Statistical Abstract of the
United States,* 1992, 112th ed.; Public Health Macroview, 1990; and the U.S. Department of
Commerce, 1993, *U.S. Industrial Outlook 1993—Health and Medical Services.*

soared 125%, the average cost of a day in the hospital rose by more than I,000% (3). Figure 5.3 illustrates where our national health care dollar was projected to be spent in fiscal I993 (5).

THE NATION'S HEALTH-CARE DOLLAR

Where it comes from:

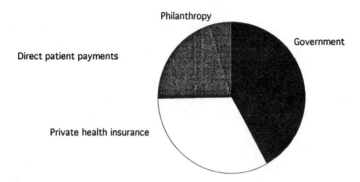

Where it goes:

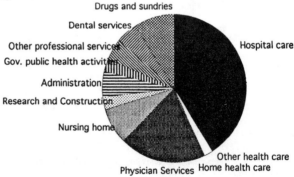

Fig. 5.3. Distribution of health expenditures by source and type of expenditure. Projection for 1993.

There are a number of reasons why health care is expensive. It is a labor intensive industry and one in which laws and practices limit the way personnel may be used. Large portions of the industry are nonprofit, e.g., Blue Cross/Blue Shield and many hospitals and other health care agencies and institutions. Technology urges us to spend money on new machines, devices, and a raft of disposables. Providers, not always the best informed persons on costs, often determine which services are to be offered. Since government, public, and private third-part reimbursement plans and not the consumer have absorbed the cost of most health care, we all tend to be less conscious of costs. Consumers are limited in their ability to "comparison shop" for health care, as they are generally not well informed about alternatives, and many people have limited or no choice due to their health insurance plan. When people are well they do not like to think about being ill. Consequently, they do not investigate the institutions in their community. There also continues to be "no unified consumer movement in health care in this country" (4). Physicians, hospitals, managed care providers such as HMOs, and nursing home chains have a virtual monopoly on services. And finally, groups like the American Medical Association are influential in limiting the numbers of those who may be prepared as professional providers.

To put things in perspective, however, it is important to point out that Americans continue to spend significantly more on such items as tobacco, eating out, personal care, and recreation than on health (6).

Interestingly, the client's share of health care costs as out-of-pocket payments has declined from 67.5% in 1950 of total private expenditures to 36.3% in 1990. In the same period, the share of private insurance and government (see Figure 5.4) as third-party payers has increased to 76.7% of every health dollar in 1990. Per capita spending appears in Figure 5.5).

Federal health care dollars are spent primarily for Medicare and Medicaid, with the remainder of the budget going, in descending order, for food and nutrition programs, pollution control, VA hospital care, health research and education, miscellaneous health care programs, prevention and control, and health planning and construction (6). State health expenditures appear in Figure 5.6.

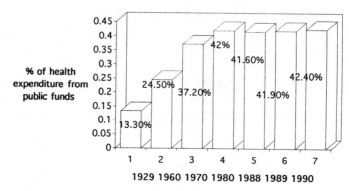

Fig. 5.4. Public spending as expressed by percent of total spending.

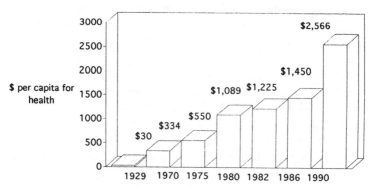

Fig. 5.5. Per capita expenditures for health care.

Hospital care continues to head the list for health care costs, followed by professional services, nursing home care, drugs, administration, insurance, other services, dental services, public health activities, other personal health care, research and development, vision products, home health care, and construction (5). Sadly, while hospital care expenditures have increased outrageously, expenditures for prevention programs have not increased.

Close to 213 million Americans have some health insurance under private or public programs (10). Unfortunately, this coverage is usually far from all-inclusive. Nearly a fifth of those insured are not covered for medical (physician) services in hospitals; many are not

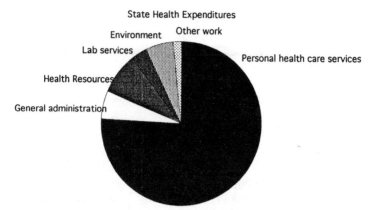

Fig. 5.6 Spending by states for health care

covered for care which takes place in ambulatory settings, for visits to other health care providers, or for prescription drugs (6,7,11). Most plans have deductibles, specify the portion the policy holder must pay, and/or limit benefits in total amount per calendar year or per number of hospital days. Premium rates have skyrocketed, there is often a waiting period for coverage to begin, and non-group premiums are prohibitively expensive. Since dental insurance became available, private insurance pays for about 34% of expenses; out-of-pocket payments are 56%.

Those who fall between the cracks for private insurance or the "Blues" are those who cannot afford premiums for individual (versus group) membership—the self-employed, part-time workers, or those working for a company that has no health plan. With escalating premiums, some employees find themselves unable to afford health insurance even when it is available. Companies with fewer than 100 employees are the least likely to offer insurance. Moreover, persons with chronic diseases, serious health problems, or functional limitations may be ineligible for coverage by the "Blues" or private insurance (13). It is interesting to note that 2.3% of registered nurses have no health insurance and most health care workers in low paying jobs have none. Of clerical workers, 7.3% have no health insurance; for laundry workers and housekeepers, the rate is 14.5%; for aides, 19.8%; and for food service workers, 20%. (37).

In this chapter, Blue Cross/Blue Shield, federal programs, private insurance, health maintenance organizations, and other managed care options will be explored in relation to the contribution of each to health care delivery.

Private Health Insurance

First on the scene to provide some assistance with health care costs were the private insurance companies. In 1847, a Boston company organized a plan for paying medical costs (8, p. 93). Over a century ago, mining, construction, and lumber companies began to employ physicians to care for their employees, who paid for the health care through small deductions from their pay (9, pp. 149-150). The Depression provided some impetus for more groups to begin similar plans, but the surge of growth came after World War II. Labor unions then began to bargain for health insurance coverage as an employment benefit (8, p. 93).

Today, there are some 1,500 private commercial insurance companies that have benefit arrangements for health or illness care for some 106 million Americans (10,12). The 12 largest companies control about 60% of the industry. These same huge companies are in the life insurance business. They exert great political influence capable of affecting the direction of national health insurance legislation. These companies, which operate largely through group employee plans, offer hospital and some outpatient/physician care. Some extended care or catastrophic plans are also available for coverage beyond that which basic plans provide (10).

Some insurance plans actually increase costs of care because they encourage and/or will pay only for more expensive hospital care as opposed to outpatient care. Most plans have coverage that is significantly better or exclusively for inpatient services (15). Commercial insurance, too, may pay only a stipulated amount for service, even if the cost is significantly higher. The role of private commercial companies is still a significant one in our health care system. In order to understand policies, some common health insurance terms are defined in Table 5.2. Table 5.1 compares Blue Cross/Blue Shield and commercial health insurance.

Table 5.1   A Comparison of Blue Cross/Blue Shield and Commercial Health Insurance.

Blue Cross/Blue Shield	Commercial Health Insurance
Health insurance their only business	Monoline companies have health insurance their only business; most health insurance plans come out of casualty companies
Payment to providers	Cash to the insured and/or providers
Group experience rated	Experience rated
Contracts based on risks	Contracts based on risks
Deals with physicians, hospitals—pays the provider of services	Deals directly with the insured; cash payments to policy holder but may reimburse providers
Nonprofit	Established for profit
Some deductibles	Some deductibles
Co-insurance	Co-insurance
Limitations on coverage	Limitations on coverage
Group (80+%) and individual plans	Group (75%) and individual plans; group self-insurance—commercial companies may be administrators for for plans
Blue Cross: hospitalization insurance. Blue Shield: in-hospital physician services; limited office, some dental and prescription drugs; Medigap policies	Hospitalization insurance: in-hospital physician services, limited office, some dental and prescription drugs; disability insurance and long-term care insurance also available; Medigap policies for Medicare eligible persons.
Some group major medical policies	Major medical policies; cash payment policies
Rates supervised and monitored by state insurance commissioner	Supervised by state insurance commissioner; no rate regulation except that rate be high enough to cover claims.

Table 5.1 (Continued)

Blue Cross/Blue Shield	Commercial Health Insurance
Benefits measured in units of service	Benefits measured in cash amounts
Can invest premium monies >90% of money taken in returned	Can invest premium monies <90% of money taken-in returned
Exempt from state premium taxes in most states	May incur state premium taxes
Insure <50% of Americans covered by insurance	Insure >50% of Americans covered by insurance
Service benefits, Blue Shield usually indemnity	Indemnity benefits
Exempt from federal taxes	Subject to federal corporate taxes
Promise of service to the community	Commercial company--motive is profit
Regulated by department or commissioner of insurance in most states	Stock or mutual companies regulated by the department or commissioner of insurance in all states
Proposed increase in rates must be filed in some states	Proposed rate increases must be filed in all states
Boards of directors dominated by hospital representatives	Boards of directors include founders or representatives of their interests
Operating expenses: 67 Blue Cross, 68 Blue Shield	Operating expenses: more than 1,500 commercial companies
Strive for success of member hospitals and physicians	Strive to generate a surplus in order to pay dividends to shareholders

Table 5.2   Glossary of Health Insurance Terms*

Out-of-pocket payment. The amount a client must pay for health services; the cost the client is responsible for.

Prepayment. The paying in advance for health care, as in an HMO.

Deductible. The amount of money that an insured person must pay for health care before insurance will pay anything at all.

Coinsurance or copayment. The percent of total cost of a particular service that the person pays out-of-pocket; for example, 25% of of a hospital room. Copayment refers to the small out-of-pocket payment fee the client must pay; $1 per visit to a physician or clinic.

Risk. The chance of losing or making money that an insurance company computes for a group or individual.

Fee-for-service. Payment by an insurance company or a client, patient, or government to a provider of care. The fee is set by the provider, not the insurance company.

Cost-plus. Payment by an insurance company or government to a provider of care for the actual cost of the services provided plus an extra amount for profit and/or administrative expenses.

Capitation. Payment by an insurance company or government to a provider of care in which the provider is paid a fixed amount of money each year per client, as in the British National Health Care system.

Premium. The monthly, quarterly, or yearly amount paid by a person to an insurance company to have a policy, or paid to an HMO or other prospective managed care plan to be enrolled.

Benefit. The amount of money paid out by an insurance company for health care services used by the policy owner. The list of services that an insurance company will pay for or that an HMO or other managed care plan will offer.

Underwriting losses. The amount of money that an insurance company pays for benefits and "administrative expenses" in excess of what it receives in premiums. The insurance company also makes money on investments, so it can have an underwriting loss and still make a profit. Usually insurance companies make up losses on health insurance with other types of insurance.

Community rating. Charging the same price for an insurance policy for each person in a community regardless of age, sex, or health condition, such as in a group plan at an industrial company.

Experience rating. Charging different prices for the same insurance policy to different people based on their age, sex, or health condition. Under experience rating, older and sicker people (who experience more health care) have to pay more for health insurance.

Table 5.2 (Continued)

Utilization. Simply means the amount of services delivered

Peer review. Attempts to control the quality of health care by having a group of providers look at a small sample of other providers' patient records to check for errors and assess the general quality of care.

Administrative expenses. Generally includes all the money that an insurance company, HMO, or other managed care provider spends for such things as salaries for executives and administrators, wages for workers, furniture and interior decoration, Muzak systems, plush carpets, office supplies, advertising, free transportation, free cars, and meals for executives on "business trips," plus other assorted fringe benefits for executives and administrators.

---

*Adapted from Billions for Band-Aids. In E. Harding, T. Bodenheimer, and S. Cummings, eds., *An Analysis of the U.S. Health Care System and of Its Reform.* San Francisco: Medical Committee for Human Rights, 1972.

Blue Cross/Blue Shield

Stepchildren of the Great Depression, the Blues, as they are known, arose out of the need for hospitals and physicians to find an alternate source of income. Many of the philanthropists who had financed nonprofit hospitals lost their investments permanently. Thus, "third party payment" of the nonprofit variety was born. The 1929 plan between Dallas teachers and Baylor Hospital was the prototype for all Blue Cross plans. The plan was sponsored by hospitals, not by commercial concerns. Subscribers received service (hospital care) in return for premiums (14, pp. 126-127). Physicians saw this system as an opportunity to guarantee their own incomes for inpatient medical care rendered and to forestall the establishment of national health insurance. Blue Shield thus came into being.

Most Blue Cross managing boards are controlled by hospital representatives. Similarly, most Blue Shield boards are composed predominantly of physicians (16). Thus, those who collect the payments also set the fees and control the administration of these nonprofit plans (16). Although public representatives on boards have increased, they usually constitute far from a majority.

Blue Cross/Blue Shield play a large role in the Medicaid and Medicare programs. The Blues were chosen as administrators for both federal Medicare and state Medicaid. Their functions are multidimensional: determining provider reimbursement, handling the reimbursement for services rendered, auditing books of the providers, and playing a significant role in utilization review. In recent years, however, the dominant role of the Blues has been eroded, and in some states private insurance companies are the administrators and also the carriers for Medicare Part B (50).

Blue Cross/Blue Shield, as well as commercial plans, have begun to include some benefits for dental care, outpatient care, nursing home services, skilled nursing care, and prescription drugs. However, as services increase, so do premium rates. In spite of the large numbers of person covered by commercial or nonprofit insurance, the government today pays the largest proportion of health care costs.

Blue Cross and Blue Shield still represent insurance for illness care and are still very much hospital oriented. Since commercial companies are numerous, the Blues have traditionally dominated health insurance in most states and thus, in many cases, health policy as well. However, that has changed with the advent of managed care models, the growth of HMOs, and power of employers as purchasers of health care benefit packages. The influence of hospitals and the Blues are eroding rapidly in our changing health care system.

Medicaid/Medicare

It became obvious, after the inception of Blue Cross/Blue Shield and commercial insurance plans, that there were still many Americans not covered for their health care needs. The fabric of the private health insurance blanket, woven in the 1930s to appease supporters of the national health insurance plan that was originally part of the Social Security Act, had worn very thin in many places. The moths of inflation, unemployment, retirement, part-time employment, deductibles, coinsurance, risk, and lack of coverage had all but eaten away the big blue blanket.

Thus it was that in 1965 Medicaid and Medicare, Title 19 and Title 18 of the Social Security Amendment, were born (14, p. 164). Table 5.3 is an attempt to distinguish the characteristics of each of these.

Table 5.3   A Comparison of Medicare and Medicaid

Medicare Title XVIII	Medicaid Title XIX
Amendment to Social Security Act 1965	Amendment to Social Security Act 1965
Hospitalization insurance for the aged and permanently disabled	Grants to states for Medical Assistance Programs
Administered at the federal levels through the Social Security Administration	Administered at federal, state, and local levels (50 different programs)
Financed by payroll tax paid by employees and employers under FICA. Part B by monthly premiums and federal government	Financed by cost-sharing between the federal government and the state
Eligibility: all persons 65 and older and certain disabled persons	Eligibility varies state to state: includes institutionalized elders, poor elders, individuals on welfare under AFDC, Supplemental Security Income (SSI) for blind, disabled, and the medically indigent; children and certain pregnant women
Part A: hospitalization (paid by payroll tax): skilled nursing facility following hospitalization, home health care, hospice care; Part B: physician's services (monthly premium); medical supplies, long-term care—private insurance, home health care, outpatient hospital services, some drugs; catastrophic (monthly premiums)	
Coverage mandated by federal government	Certain services mandated by federal government; program design and benefits left to individual states
Over 90% of those 65 and older eligible	Eligibility left to states—estimates of millions with incomes below the poverty level who are not eligible

Table 5.3   (Continued)

Medicare Title XVIII	Medicaid Title XIX
2/3 of federal expenditures on health pay less than 1/2 of the health bills of older adults	Much of the total U.S. Medicaid bill spent in only a few states
Major expenditures for hospitalization—limited, annual deductible, cost-sharing	Major expenditures for nursing home and intermediate care facilities, then hospital care
Co-insurance and deductibles, balance billing by physician	Virtually no co-insurance, but benefits vary considerably from state to state
Free choice of provider	Free choice of provider, but limited to those willing to take Medicaid clients
Prospective payment system in place (DRGs)	Prospective payment system
Some contracting with HMOs for Part B	Some contracting with HMOs

Medicare

The politics involved in the passage of the Medicare bill represent a long historical struggle between those original supporters of the national health insurance plan which was amputated from the Social Security Act of the 1930s and powerful lobby groups such as American Medical Association. The original Medicare proposal was made in 1952; Congress did not exhibit serious concern with the problems of the elderly until 1958, and then it took seven years of finance committee hearings before the Medicare bill was finally passed (16).

Medicare is financed under the Social Security Administration. Some of the funds come from federal revenues, but most come from employee payroll deductions. Medicare provides hospital, some nursing home care, and some home care services for citizens 65 years of age and more. By paying a monthly fee, a person can enroll in Part B, voluntary supplementary medical insurance (SMI), and receive, in addition, some physician, outpatient, and medical supplies coverage. The premium for Part B has increased steadily since its inception. For older Americans on fixed incomes, the deductibles and premiums may be out of reach.

Medicare is administered under 50 private and local Blue Cross/Blue Shield organizations and several other independent organizations which act as "fiscal intermediaries." They determine benefits, make payments, and audit the records of providers (10).

In 1972, amendments were passed allowing disabled persons under 65 and those never covered by Social Security, many of whom were women and farm laborers, to enroll in Medicare. However, these persons have to pay monthly premiums for both Part A and Part B. This amendment also mandates a local utilization review board (16).

In 1983, legislation was passed and implemented which mandated prospective payment under Medicare for hospital care, using 468 diagnosis-related groups (DRGs) for rate setting and to set length of stay. Thus, when a person is admitted, the admitting diagnosis determines when he/she will be discharged (17, p. 697). A study of the financial impact of variability in resource use within the DRG prospective payment system showed that DRGs must be adjusted for severity of illness and that homogeneity of case mix groups is important to an equitable system. Thus refinements in the system need to continue to be made as the prospective system continues in use with Medicare clients and is extended to other sources of reimbursement and other settings (18). The DRG system does not offer nurses the opportunity to build a data base to predict use of nursing resources (19, p. 438). DRGs also create ethical dilemmas for nurses because of the fixed length of hospital stays and limited coverage by Medicare for home care services (20).

The fallout for nursing from DRGs has been multifaceted. In addition to sicker patients in hospitals, patients are discharged sicker, placing new responsibilities on those who provide home care. It is not uncommon for patients to be home on intravenous drips, respirators, and other high technology equipment. More services and more nursing hours are required, and providers are less able to refer patients to hospitals or to other health care professionals (38, 39). Inadequacies in long-term care reimbursement have become more evident; not only do more persons require long-term care, but they are sicker and need more services (40).

Since the institution of DRGs for Medicare patients, numerous studies have been done to examine the impact of the universal application of the system. Many of these studies have emphasized the need that hospitals have to balance revenues with expenses. When hospitals handling trauma cases are included in studies of costs and DRGs, for example, revenue losses are staggering, because of the costs of caring for the critically injured (41). Some states have experimented with DRGs for Medicaid patients as well, demonstrating reduced rates of increase in spending for hospitalization (42). Private managed care systems, including HMOs and PPOs (preferred provider organizations) have instituted incentives to shorten lengths of stay for patients, using in essence the DRG system.

In the decades since Medicare was instituted, older adults have fared rather poorly. In 1991, they were spending over $67 billion for health care out-of-pocket, compared to $17.5 billion in 1961, before Medicare was enacted. A major portion of these expenses goes for nursing home costs, not covered by Medicare (Medicare pays only 4.7% of nursing home costs nationwide). Insurance premiums have also risen dramatically, as four of five elderly obtain Medigap policies to cover Medicare cost-sharing requirements. Medicare Part B premiums have risen as well (21). Medigap policies became a new gold mine for private insurance companies in the 1980s. as cost-sharing in Medicare escalated. In 1990, Congress enacted legislation to prohibit abusive practices and require adherence to strict standards for policies (43). In 1988, recognizing that poor seniors and persons with disabilities could not pay out-of-pocket expenses related to Medicare, Congress enacted legislation known as buy-in (officially, the Qualified Medicare Beneficiary Program—QMB). This requires state Medicaid programs to pay the Medicare premiums and deductibles for those with incomes below the federal poverty line (44).

Medicaid

Medicaid was passed along with Medicare in 1965. There the similarity essentially ends. It is a health care program for the poor and is paid for out of federal, state, and some local funds.

One of Medicaid's purposes was to remove the "tiered" approach to health care services. Those who could not pay for services had been labeled "charity patients" for whom doctors and hospitals provided free care. These were the people often used as guinea pigs for experiments and for training health care providers.

Medicaid was to eliminate all this inequality. The program is administered individually by each of the 50 states. The general purpose of the bill is to provide assistance for medical care for families with dependent children, for the disabled, and for all those with insufficient funds to obtain care not covered under special Social Security Insurance (SSI) benefits. Rehabilitation is to be included in the services (22, p. 57). Eligibility determination is left up to each state. In addition, the general guidelines are so broad that each state interprets what services are to be covered. Of course, each state has to submit a plan to the Department of Health and Human Services for approval. Since it is a program with matching federal funds, considerable control can be exerted by Health and Human Services if it chooses to do so.

Coverage includes basic services for hospitalization, outpatient hospital care, laboratory and x-ray studies, nursing home care for those over 21, and physician services (22, pp. 65-66). Payments go directly to providers.

States can, in addition, opt to include other services for which federal matching funds are available. These include home health care, dental care, prescription drugs, eyeglasses, orthopedic devices, private duty nurses, physical therapy, nursing home care for persons over 65 in a tuberculosis or mental institution, and any other services approved by the Secretary of the Department of Health and Human Services (22, p. 66). Thus, wealthy states have many options, whereas other states struggle to provide the basic mandated services.

Unlike Medicare, all funds for Medicaid come out of general federal and state revenues. Spending in 1990 ranged from $1,444 per recipient in West Virginia to $5,100 in New York (26). Benefits are supposedly unlimited, but may be limited because of funds; there is rarely a coinsurance clause. Hospitals are reimbursed for costs and provider charges on a fee basis. Because Medicaid fees are often lower than those for Medicare, 44 states have major problems getting physicians to participate in Medicaid (45).

In 1990, only 45.2% of people under the federal poverty line were covered: 39.2% of white persons below the poverty level, 57.8% of Blacks, 44.7% of Latinos, 61.9% of those under 18 (6). At the same time, the number of Americans, especially children, living in poverty is rising (46). Income levels for eligibility for Medicaid are often unreasonable. Eligibility and residence requirements exclude many, among them migrant farm workers and many rural Americans. Moreover, as with Medicare, Medicaid does not ensure access or availability of services. Thus, even when coverage is provided, many people cannot get to health care facilities or the facilities are nonexistent. Escalating costs have necessitated cuts in coverage and virtual elimination of some elective care. Between 1980 and 1989, serious erosion of maternal and child health under Medicaid occurred, and the rate (22%) of children living in poverty is now the highest in 20 years (48).

In 1988, legislation was passed by Congress to expand coverage to groups previously not covered: children and pregnant women with household incomes that do not exceed 185% of the federal poverty line, and children ages 5 to 8 in households that do not exceed 100% of the poverty line (36).

Congress passed the Omnibus Budget Reconciliation Act of 1990, including a phased-in mandatory eligibility for children in families below the federal poverty level and continuation of eligibility for pregnant women and infants. States continued to address problems of eligibility for their uninsured citizens. Minnesota, Florida, and Vermont passed bills to ensure coverage for all, incorporating Medicaid programs into their plans, and several states experimented with managed care models for Medicaid recipients (49). Numerous states have passed Child Health Insurance Reform Plans (CHIRP) mandating coverage of preventive services for children; these incorporate Medicaid eligible children, and mandate insurers doing business in those states to provide such coverage. In 1993, states were assured of full federal financial participation if they wished to expand Medicaid income eligibility to children and pregnant women (47).

Health Maintenance Organizations (HMOs)

Health Maintenance organizations are not a new concept, although legislation for planning them is fairly recent (1971). The Mayo Clinic, begun in 1887 by the brothers Mayo, evolved into the first large-scale group practice; from it the health maintenance organization concept evolved.

In 1929, a Farmer's Union Cooperative Health Association was founded in Oklahoma. The oldest large-scale prepaid plan in this country is the Kaiser-Permanente program, established over 40 years ago. Henry Kaiser, an industrialist, in association with a physician, Sidney Garfield, set up a prepaid group practice for his workers on the Hoover Dam project. After World War II, the plan was opened to the public (24, pp. 4-5). Today there are over 2,500 nurses working in the nine major Kaiser medical centers in California alone. Kaiser-Permanente is the largest HMO in the country, with an enrollment of over six million members across the U.S. (25).

An HMO may be a group of physicians, a prepaid health cooperative, or a comprehensive health insurance plan developed by an organization such as an industry (e.g., Connecticut General), an insurance company, a medical school, or Blue Cross/Blue Shield, e.g. Rhode Island Group Health, now part of the Harvard Community Health Plan (HCHP) HMO system (26). The idea is to contract for delivery of health services, offer comprehensive benefits (both inpatient and ambulatory), draw on a voluntary target population which may include groups and/or individuals, and elicit prepayment from each enrolled member. The emphasis is on primary care and health maintenance, since health care costs are less if people are kept well. Studies have shown that HMO patients are hospitalized less often and, when hospitalized, have shorter stays than patients covered by other types of plans (26).

It has been estimated that it takes some two million dollars or more to set up an HMO; that a target group of at least 20,000 clients is necessary; and that a period of two to four years of operation is needed to break even.

There are four HMO models currently: (1) an HMO can contract with physicians for its members (Independent Practice Association—IPA); (2) an HMO can contract with one or more groups (IPAs) in different geographic areas; (3) a group practice of physicians can provide care at one or more sites; (4) an HMO can be one or more centers—all providers are employees; this is known as a group HMO. (26)

Proponents argue that HMOs offer no financial incentive for unnecessary services and that they eliminate unnecessary hospitalization and cut costs. Opponents hold that is socialized medicine, that it is assembly line medicine, that care is mediocre, that there is skimping on personpower and services, and that often no system is provided to monitor quality of care. In addition, it has been argued that such plans tend to cut out those who are poor, elderly, or chronically ill, and that thus cost figures are deceptive. By 1989, however, 27 states were experimenting with HMO enrollment for Medicaid recipients (24). HMOs are also used for Medicare and CHAMPUS patients. Some incentives have encouraged HMOs to enter competition for Medicare clients, and the Health Care Financing Administration (HCFA) has encouraged enrollment of persons eligible for Medicaid in HMOs (26.)

Legislation

In 1971, legislation was passed providing monies for investigating the cost effectiveness of HMOs for Medicaid recipients and for developing such programs (27). In 1973, the Health Maintenance Organization Act was passed. This bill provided financial assistance for establishing HMOs. It protected the right of citizens to choose an HMO or alternative mode of care when both were available. It also overrode restrictive state laws where they existed (28). The bill also legislated the requirements for an HMO. By l982, however, Congress had all but eliminated such funds.

It is too soon to measure the overall impact of HMOs on health care. Their number is increasing rapidly. Eager to get into the arena, Blue Cross and private insurance companies have begun HMOs, as have many companies who are using the concept for their employee health benefits. By l991, there were 556 operational HMOs or individual practice associations (IPAs) in the United States serving 34.1 million people compared with l75 in l976 serving six million people (6). Of these, 208 were group HMOs and 348 were IPAs.

Other Managed Care Models

Several models exist for managed care in addition to HMOs. Preferred Provider Organizations (PPOs) contract with networks of health care providers who agree to provide services for fees within a negotiated fee schedule. Members can choose care from a non-affiliated provider, but pay a financial penalty. Exclusive PPOs do not allow any care outside the network unless the person chooses to pay out-of-pocket for the care. Finally, Point-of-Service Plans (POSs) are a combination of an HMO and PPO, using a network of care providers. Each member chooses a primary care provider who in turn makes all specialty referrals. Out of plan providers can be used, but the member pays higher deductibles and co-payments (10).

Toward the Future: Nursing and Cost Containment

Some interesting studies are emerging directed toward reducing health care costs. One of these, which looks at the roles of nurses in advanced practice, is most promising (30). It documents the cost-effectiveness and quality of care provided by nurse-midwives and nurse practitioners. Nurses, after all, are frequently those with whom clients have the most contact in clinics, hospitals, and other health care delivery settings. Additionally, nurses are recognized in the community as providers and educators in schools, senior centers, visiting nurse agencies, public health agencies, and neighborhood health centers.

As of 1989, there were approximately 95 nurse practitioner programs being conducted in this country (31, 34). Many nurses enrolled in these will serve as primary care providers and thus be able to provide primary care if that is the direction health care reform takes.

The bills passed in recent years in some states to reimburse nurses directly for care to clients are important steps in obtaining third-party reimbursement for all nurses as independent health care providers (35).

Since health care costs have escalated, consumers have become more aware of and vociferous about quality of care (32). Nurses must be prepared to be accountable for the care we provide, both for its quality and its cost effectiveness. Greater sensitivity to costs of day-to-day care, equipment, and services will help nurses establish our roles both as consumer advocates and as proponents of cost containment. At the same time, we must be cognizant of attempts to sacrifice quality for cost and be prepared to justify staffing patterns and the need of professional nursing care. Finally, we must speak with one voice "if nursing is going to be a force for positive change" (32, p. 130). Only when our own house is in order can we afford to criticize other providers, hospitals, or health care industries for having contributed to overall escalation of costs.

References

1. Milio, N. (1981). Promoting Health Through Public Policy. Philadelphia: F.A. Davis.
2. Grace, H. (1990). Can health care costs be contained? Nursing & Health Care 11(3):125.
3. Public Affairs Advisory. (1987). Cost Containment. New York: National League for Nursing. P. 1.
4. Annas, G.J. (1975). The Rights of Hospital Patients: The Basic American Civil Liberties Handbook. New York: Avon Books. P. 4.
5. Department of Health, Human Services, PHS, Health Care Financing Administration, 1993.
6. Statistical Abstract of the United States. (1992), 112th ed. Washington, DC: Department of Commerce, Bureau of the Census.
7. Short, P., Monheit, A.K., Beauregard, K. (1989). A Profile of Uninsured Americans. National Medical Expenditures Survey Research Findings 1. Rockville, MD: Public Health Service.

8. Schorr, D. (1970). Don't Get Sick in America. Nashville: Aurora.
9. Klaw, S. (1975). The Great American Medicine Show. New York: Penguin.
10. Source Book of Health Insurance Data 1991. (1991). Washington, DC: Health Insurance Association of America.
11. Hahn, B. and Lefkowitz, D. (1991). Annual expenses and sources of payment for health care services. National Medical Expenditure Survey Research Findings 14. Rockville, MD: Public Health Service.
12. Peck, P. (1992, January). Health care spending soared in 80's. Health Care Professional, p. 3.
13. Beauregard, K. (1991). Persons denied private insurance due to poor health. National Medical Expenditure Survey Data and Summary 4. Rockville, MD: Public Health Service.
14. Ehrenreich, J. and Ehrenreich, B. (1970). The American Health Empire: Power, Profits, and Politics. New York: Vintage.
15. Allukian, M. (1993). Forging the future: The public health imperative. American Journal of Public Health 83(5):655-660.
16. Marmor, T.R. (1973). The Politics of Medicare. Chicago: Aldine. P.23.
17. Prospective reimbursement to be in effect this year for Medicare (1983). American Journal of Nursing 83(5):697, 710.
18. Horn, S.D., Sharkey, P.D., Chambers, A.F. and Horn, R.A. (1985). Severity of illness within DRGs: Impact on prospective payment. American Journal of Public Health 75(10):1195-1199.
19. Thompson, J.D. and Diers, D. (1985). DRGs and nursing intensity. Nursing & Health Care 6(8):435-439.
20. Dupre, L. (1987). Ethical nursing and DRGs. California Nurse 10:3.
21. Elderly American are spending a much larger share of income on health than before Medicare.(1992, July). ASAP:1-5.
22. Stevens, R. and Stevens, R. (1974). Welfare Medicine in America. New York: The Free Press.
23. Medicaid inequity. (1987). The Nation's Health 17(7):5.
24. Merritt, R. (1987). State Medicaid costs up 9 percent. The Nation's Health 17(3):6.
25. Seitz, R. (1992, Dec. 20). The political tea leaves point to medical networks. The New York Times, p. 10.
26. Drew, J.C. (1990). Health maintenance organizations: History, evolution and survival. Nursing & Health Care 11(3):145-149.
27. Hughes, P.S. (1974). Medicaid's answer for better service: HMOs. Social and Rehabilitation Record 1(2):10-12.
28. Prussin, J.A. (1974). Health Maintenance Organization Legislation in 1973-74. Washington, DC: Science and Health Publications. P. 11.
29. American Nurses Association. (1981). Facts about Nursing 80-81. New York: American Journal of Nursing Company.
30. Safriet, B.J. (1992). Health care dollars and regulatory sense: The role of advanced practice nursing. Yale Journal on Regulation 9:417-488.

31. National League for Nursing. (1992). Nursing Data Review 1992. New York: NLN.
32. Grace, H. (1990). Can health costs be contained? Nursing & Health Care II(3):124-130.
33. Grimaldi, P.L. (1987). Inching toward prospective payment for outpatient hospital care. Nursing Management 18(8):26-28.
34. American Nurses Association. (1989). Directory of Accredited Organizations and Continuing Education Certificate Programs Preparing Nurse Practitioners. Kansas City, MO: American Nurses Association.
35. Pearson, L.J. (1993). Update: How each state stands on legislative issues affecting advanced nursing practice. The Nurse Practitioner 18(1):23-28, 30-32, 35-36, 38.
36. Medicaid eligibility expanded. (1988). Child Health Financing Report 5(2):1.
37. Himmelstein, D.U. and Woolhandler, S. (1991, July 17). Who cares for the caregivers? Journal of the American Medical Association, 399-401.
38. Phillips, E.K., Fisher, M.E., MacMillan-Scattergood, D. and Baglioni, A.J. (1989). DRG ripple and the shifting burden of care to home care. Nursing & Health Care 10(6):325-327.
39. Wood, J.B. and Estes, C.L. (1990). The impact of DRGs on community-based service providers: Implications for the elderly. American Journal of Public Health 80(7):840-843.
40. Rantz, M.J. (1990). Inadequate reimbursement for long-term care. Nursing & Health Care 11(9):470-472.
41. Mackenzie, E.J., Steinwachs, D.M. and Ramsey, A.I. (1991). Trauma case mix and hospital payment: The potential for refining DRGs. Health Services Research 26(1):5-26.
42. Hellinger, F.J. (1986). Reimbursement under diagnosis-related groups: The Medicaid experience. Health Care Financing Review 8(2):35-44.
43. Medigap changes represent victory for consumers. (1992). ASAP 8(3):1.
44. Still secret: The QMB program. (1992, July). ASAP, Special Report 1-6.
45. Pear, R. (1991, April 2). Low Medicaid fees seen as depriving the poor of care. The New York Times, A1, 14.
46. Five Million Children: 1992 Update. (1992). New York: Columbia University School of Public Health, National Center for Children in Poverty.
47. Reports of Medicaid programs, state activities in reform. (1991, 1992, 1993). Child Health Financing Report 8(2): U (1, 2, 3).
48. Cohen, S.S. (1990). The politics of Medicaid:1980-1989. Nursing Outlook 38(5):229-233.
49. Kreiger, J.W., Connell, F.A. and LoGerfo, J.P. (1992). Medicaid prenatal care: A comparison of use and outcomes in fee-for-service and managed care. American Journal of Public Health 82:185-190.
50. The Medicare 1993 Handbook. (1993). Baltimore, MD: Health Care Financing Administration.

6

Providers in the Health Care Delivery System

"In health care, the individual has been replaced by a team of specialists who individually often do not know what the others are doing"(1).

What began as an informal and simple system of health care delivery in this country some 350 years ago has burgeoned into a complexity of specialization almost beyond the comprehension of even the most sophisticated health personpower resources administrator. The simple system consisting of the medicine man, the "granny" lay midwife, and the general practitioner now exists only in remote rural areas and among those enjoying a rebirth of the lay health care movement. In just over 200 years since the founding of the first American medical school at the University of Pennsylvania, and 100 years since the first nursing schools were begun (2), the health personpower pool has become a potpourri of specialized jobs and services. There is little cause to wonder why consumers of health care are often bewildered when trying to decide whom to consult and what services to expect.

Health Personpower: USA

The health care industry is the third largest employer in the United States in terms of personpower. More than two dozen occupations in the health field are licensed in one or more states. More than ten million persons make their living in health care professsions and occupations (3, 4). The Bureau of Labor Statistics projects growth in health services industries between 1990 and 2005 at 44% (5).

Allied health personnel (aides, orderlies, ward clerks, technicians, and others who are not considered to be professionals) comprise almost two million providers. Their levels of education range from less than elementary school to college graduate (3, 4). Some have graduate degrees and are employed as allied health workers because they are unable to find employment in their particular fields. This is one of the fastest growing occupational groups in the United States (3). At the turn of the century, about 80% of health care workers were physicians. That figure now approaches 6% of the health personpower labor force (3).

Distribution of Health Personpower

One of the major problems in health care delivery in the United States is maldistribution of health care workers. As the population has shifted from rural to urban areas, the majority of health care providers has clustered in the large cities. This phenomenon has rendered some urban centers virtually saturated with providers. It should be noted, however, that maldistribution exists even within large metropolitan areas; slums may be woefully lacking in health care personnel, whereas areas with university medical centers, upper and middle class suburbs, and bedroom communities support high ratios of professionals.

In 1982, U.S. medical schools were producing about 16,000 graduate physicians a year (6). The Graduate Medical Education National Advisory committee in 1980 forecast a surplus of 70,000 physicians by 1990 (7). By 1988, however, enrollments were down (15) and only have risen again in the past couple of years. One of the problems in maldistribution and physician shortages is that most physicians choose specialties rather than primary care.

Maldistribution is blatantly apparent from figures delineating the distribution of health care professionals. In 1990 there was a mean of 216 physicians per 100,000 population. The mean number of dentists was 59 per 100,000. For nurses in 1989, the mean number was 676 per 100,000 (4). A substantial number of the rural counties in the country have no health care professionals whatever. About 89 percent of the municipalities in the United States have a population of 10,000 or less, and many of the smallest are unable to attract even one physician. Small communities often resort to advertising and entice-ments to try to attract physicians (4).

In the 1990s, 2,082 areas of the United States representing about 35 million people were designated as critical areas due to shortages of primary health care providers. These areas are designat-ed by the federal government as HPSHs (health professional shortage areas) (53). The number of physicians now ranges from a high of 334 per 100,000 to 125 per 100,000. For dentists, the range is 76 to 81 per 100,000. Similar figures can be cited for optometrists, pharmacists, chiropractors, dental hygienists, podiatrists, radiologic technicians, and veterinarians. Registered nurses range from 1,153 to 430 per 100,000 persons. New England has the highest ratio of registered nurses to population in the country, while the U.S. South has the lowest (4).

There is also a maldistribution of the more than 1.8 million allied health personnel in our country. The direct impact of this fact on health care is not as marked since these persons generally work under the direction of medical professionals (4).

Education for Health Care Providers

Today, persons desiring a career in health care delivery are confront-ed with dozens of categories of jobs, over 400 areas of specialization, five major levels of educational institutions, and a system of prepara-tion that often separates the academic from the experiential.

Education of physicians in this country began with apprenticeships and migrated to the university in the eighteenth century with the opening of the first medical school at the University of Pennsylvania. Nursing education, which began in 1873 with the founding of three hospital diploma schools based on the Nightingale model, began to move into university settings during the second decade of the twentieth century (10).

Five major levels of educational preparation now exist for those who comprise our health worker and professional labor force. Nonprofessionals or allied health personnel may receive their preparation in a nonacademic setting, usually the institution in which they are employed. They are our nurses' aides, orderlies, mental health aides, attendants, and so on. Licensed practical nurses may receive their preparation either in a nonacademic setting such as a hospital school or in a technical high school or a program at a community college. (Community colleges are preparing a wide variety of health care providers including licensed practical/vocational nurses, laboratory assistants, respiratory therapists, dental technicians and hygienists, and physical therapy aides.) Two-year associate degree programs which prepare persons to qualify for registered nurse licensing examinations are now providing an increasing number of nurses seeking registration.

Baccalaureate preparation provides education for professional practice in fields such as nursing, physical and occupational therapy, laboratory technology, clinical dietetics, and pre-professional programs for dentists, physicians, osteopaths, social workers, clinical psychologists, anthropologists, speech therapists, and so on. Postbaccalaureate education is necessary for the practice of medicine, dentistry, clinical psychology, and sometimes social work and nursing. Physical and occupational therapy and social work are moving toward requiring a master's degree for entry level practice.

The plethora of programs allowing a candidate to sit for board examinations in nursing is but one example of the confusion which has beset the process of educating health care providers. Registered nurses may have graduated from a hospital-based two- or three-year diploma program, a two-year private of community college program, a four- or five-year baccalaureate program, and may, in addition, possess a master's or doctoral degree. Any of these may be the first preparation in nursing.

The diversity and disparity among programs, degrees, and levels of preparation for careers in health provision also are factors that hinder the implementation of a team approach in health care delivery. To implement such an approach would require an educational system that encourages and fosters collaboration and mutual respect among professionals and allied health workers. There have been some attempts to establish this kind of system, e.g., by offering core programs for health care providers in universities with a number of pre-professional and professional programs. In community colleges with one-year and associate degree programs for a variety of health careers, students may take core courses together. Such efforts represent at least an initial attempt to improve communication and cooperation among health care providers for optimal health care delivery.

The Role of Government in Providing Health Care Personpower

Government involvement in support of health care personpower training has been sporadic, inconsistent, and, at times, conspicuously absent. The beginning can be traced to some of the provisions in the Social Security Act of 1935.

From its inception in 1918, the federally funded Veterans Administration hospital system has played an important role in the preparation of health care personnel through provision of clinical laboratory experiences.

In the 1960s, a number of Congressional bills were passed allocating federal monies for health personpower training. The 1963 Health Profession Education Assistance Act allocated monies for loans for students of medicine, osteopathy, podiatry, public health, pharmacy and dentistry. In 1964, the act was amended to include optometry students, and in that year the Nurse Training Act was passed. In 1966, Congress passed the Veterinary Medicine Education Act (12). Also in 1966, the Allied Health Professions and Personnel

Training Act was passed, and in 1968 the Health Manpower Act was enacted. These were all important in encouraging and supporting persons to choose health careers (13).

The 1993 budget for health personpower numbered nearly 266 million dollars, with 119 million for the National Health Service Corps (8). Monies for nursing are used for preparing educators and nurse practitioners, for nurse traineeships for master's and doctoral education, and for special grants to schools for advanced training programs. There is still a shortage of nurses with graduate degrees in addition to the regional shortages of entry level nurses. After several years of decline in appropriations for training health care professionals, projections for the 1994 budget are for an increase (8).

Personpower: Women and Minorities as Providers

About 80% of all health workers are women (4). Ninety-seven percent of registered nurses are women, as are 71% of kitchen workers and food preparers in health-care settings, 89% of aides, 95% of licensed vocational and technical nurses, 94% of nutritionists, 95% of health office workers, 94% of health record technologists, 78% of clinical laboratory technologists, 98% of dental assistants, and 68% of social workers. In contrast, 83% of physicians, 90% of chiropractors, 90% of dentists, 63% of physicians' assistants, and 80% of hospital administrators are men. More than 80% of allied health workers are women clustered either in their teens or their late 30s or older (4).

Most physicians are white and most are from upper and upper middle-class families. Nurses and technicians tend to be lower middle-class, white, and female. Aides, cooks, and maids are generally lower class, African-American, Chicano, Puerto Rican, or other Hispanic.

Minority groups furnish 8.7% of medical and professional providers and anywhere from 20 to 30% or more of the various types of nonprofessionals. The proportion of minority students in medical schools has increased to more than 15.9%, and the proportion of women enrolled has more than tripled (16), and in the class graduating in 1991 was 32.2% (14, 15).

Wage differentials for jobs follow sex lines. Women make less money than men in comparable positions. Male nurses earn more than female nurses. The most important reason for the great wage differential between men and women is that "society has always assigned less value to women's work, even though it isn't inherently or necessarily any less valuable than men's work" (17). The distribution of health provider positions by sex, socioeconomic, and ethnic background, and wages forms an inverse pyramid. Relatively small numbers of white males dominate the high income professions such as medicine, dentistry, and hospital administration. Women and minorities comprise the largest number of nurses, paraprofessionals, and workers in allied health positions, and receive markedly smaller incomes. The nursing shortage of the 1980s finally forced health care agencies to raise salaries for nurses substantially (18). Average salaries of health care professionals have grown over the decade, but professions dominated by men continue to earn considerably more than those in which women are predominate.

Nursing

An Historical Look. Nursing evolved as an outgrowth of the nurturing role of women toward their children, families, and neighbors. It became an acceptable professional calling for women, akin to motherhood. Medicine was largely closed to women of the nineteenth century because they were unable to obtain the education necessary for entrance to university medical schools.

After the first U.S. nursing schools founded on the Nightingale model opened in 1873, hospital training schools erupted rapidly as the advantages of having students to provide much needed nursing care became apparent. We are still beset by the vestiges of the Victorian rules for Nightingale schools, which emphasized subservience of nurses (women) to physicians (men). The traditions of deference to male authority, the nurse's cap as a symbol of humility and obedience, and the role of mother surrogate die hard. Mrs. Fenwick, once matron of St. Bartholomew's Hospital in London, wrote in 1877 at the time of the emergence of professional nursing organizations: "The nurse question is the woman question; we shall have to run the gauntlet of those historic rotten eggs" (19).

Nursing was beginning as a profession just as the women's movement was gaining momentum. Surprisingly, there were very few nursing leaders among the radical feminists. Ashley says, "The failure of nurses to identify with radical feminists seeking to change the social order led to the failure of the nursing profession to liberate both education and practice" (20, p. 146).

The Goldmark Report's findings (21), published in 1923, were the result of an exhaustive study of nursing in the United States. Two of the report's ten recommendations were that nurse educators, nursing leaders, and public health nurses receive additional training beyond the generic programs, and that they also receive endowment funds for nursing education. This report led to the establishment of schools of nursing at Yale and Vanderbilt. The report also gave rise to the study on the grading of nursing schools undertaken by the National League for Nursing, which resulted in the closing of many inferior schools.

The Flexner report of 1910 greatly influenced the evolution of medical education and singlehandedly caused the closing of many of the medical schools then open to women and Blacks (22). Because medicine was now closed to women, many of them went into nursing.

The shortage of nurses during World War II prompted the federal government to earmark millions of dollars to assist schools in educating nurses and providing refresher courses. In addition, the United States Cadet Nurse Corps was created (23). This set the stage for later federal legislation to support nursing education. The 1963 report of the Surgeon General's Consultant Group on Nursing (24) provided much needed data on the supply of nurses and the need for federal support for education and research.

Education and the Supply of Nurses. There are approximately two million registered nurses holding active licenses to practice in the United States today, of whom about 1.5 million are employed in nursing. The majority are women (96.7%) and the majority of these are married. Some 13% are from the following minority backgrounds: African-American, 7.1%; Hispanic, 2.4%; American Indian, 0.3%,

Asian, 3% (4, 11).

The majority of employed nurses work in patient care settings, mostly hospitals (68%). Most nurses in practice continue to be prepared at the associate degree level. Many attend diploma programs, although these have declined dramatically in number over the past decade. Over half a million nurses now hold either a baccalaureate, master's, or doctoral degree (11).

Toward the end of 1986, employers began to have difficulty in hiring nurses. Schools of nursing noted a trend toward declining enrollments, and several schools of nursing across the nation had closed, in part due to the small number of students. Employers began extensive recruitment campaigns to attract nurses (25, 52).

Solutions to the shortage proposed by the American Nurses Association included: support for nursing education, primarily at the baccalaureate level, through the federal government; compensation for nurses commensurate with that of other professionals; and practice responsibilities consistent with educational preparation (28). The class of 1989 was the smallest in decades. By 1993, enrollments in nursing schools were way up, applications outpaced enrollments three to one, and nursing vacancy rates were down (54, 59).

Evolving Role of Nursing. "The role of nursing in the health field is the epitome of women's role in American society" (20, p. 125). In spite of the pitfalls associated with being a woman's profession, all too closely akin to motherhood, and one viewed by many as more of a temporary occupation than a profession, nursing has made great strides in the past century. The movement of nursing education into institutions of higher education and the recent growing support of the baccalaureate degree for entry into professional practice bring nursing closer to other health professions. The surge of programs to prepare nurses for expanded roles and the support for research strengthen professional status. Scope of practice statements and standards for practice developed by nurses secure a voice for nursing as to what nurses shall and shall not do (26, 27, 29, 30, 31, 33, 34).

Nurses have great potential for power within the health care system. The exercise of that power should be a goal for the 1990s. Nurses can "truly begin to capture the power, influence, and esteem necessary to promote improved health care for clients" (35, p. 82). This statement is as true in the 1990s as it was when it was written in 1978.

Organization of the Provider Hierarchy

There has been a dramatic shift in the organization of the medically dominated hierarchy of health care providers over the past few decades. Prior to World War II, the majority of physicians were solo practitioners and most were in general practice. Today fewer than 50% are in solo practice and only 56% give direct patient care in office practice. Specialists (88.5%) now outnumber general practitioners (11.5%) (4).

A number of factors have loosened the power grip of physicians over the whole health care delivery system. The power structure of the American Medical Association has yielded some of its clout to the "Blues" (Blue Cross and Blue Shield), to private insurers, and to professional health care administrators. The percentage of physicians who are AMA members is declining, and AMA members are increasingly dependent on hospitals and the power of the American Hospital Association (32). Creation of the National Practitioner Data Bank means that physicians barred from practice or disciplined in one state will be unable to practice in others (56). Nurses and other providers are moving toward more autonomous practice. They are also demanding a greater voice in formulating health policy. In 1992, nurses were granted a seat on the board of commissioners of the Joint Commission on Accreditation of Health Care Organizations (JCAHO) (36, 37). As health care reforms under consideration point to an emphasis on primary care, a review of the roles of advanced practice nurses underscores our abilities to deliver quality, cost-effective primary care (50).

The public is becoming vociferous in its demands for accountability, cost control, and quality of care. More emphasis is being directed toward the quality of the relationship between provider and consumer (41). Much power now lies with institutions as shifts occur in technology, the financing of health care, pressures of managed care, and the changing prestige of physicians within institutions. Collective bargaining among health care workers influences power distribution markedly. All of these factors contribute to a rapidly changing and diversified distribution of power in the health care system.

Diversity and Dissent

In the 1990s, the financial crises in our so-called health care delivery system have precipitated crises for health care professionals, particularly nurses. In efforts to save money, hospitals have renamed the registered care technicians of the 1980s "unlicensed assistive personnel (UAP)." These persons are supposed to perform non-nursing tasks. More questions than answers have arisen about these new health care providers. In some of our major cities, nurses are being laid off and replaced by UAPs (39, 40).

"Today the health professions of nursing, medicine, pharmacy, dentistry, social work, and allied fields are facing some major conflict stresses related to both professional health services and educational endeavors" (42). To this might be added the stresses of financial constraints, public outcries for health care reform, and shifts in the settings for health care delivery.

Areas of conflict include:

1. Ways to provide new and effective modes of health care delivery to meet needs of consumers.
2. Ways to be economical, socially accountable, and humanistic.
3. Ways to change health practice by using research and new ideas.
4. Ways to deal with collective bargaining.
5. Ways to retain standards from education and carry them over into practice.
6. Ways to heighten productivity and accountability.
7. Ways to deal with observations of less than desirable practice or malpractice by others (42).
8. Ways to protect ourselves and our clients from risk (56, 57).

9.   Dealing with stress (58).

Some suggestions for change include the following:

1.   Some relinquishing of professional "turf" to allow for sharing responsibility, with an emphasis on colleagueship, not competition.
2.   Participation by nurses and other health professionals in decision-making for health care.
3.   Levels of education commensurate with expected levels of performance (43).
4.   Health team approach during the educational process.
5.   Rewards within the system for humanistic, quality care, and for caring (38).
6.   Collaboration in research among disciplines.

Collective Bargaining

The amendment to the Taft-Hartley Act of 1947 (National Labor Relations Act) gives to professionals and nonprofessionals in voluntary hospitals the right to organized and bargain (44, p. 284). This amendment has profound implications for the model in which the sole authority rests in the hands of physicians (45). It also has important implications for maintenance of control by professionals over standards of practice. Nurses have begun to recognize that in certain institutions the exercise of their legal right to bargain collectively and to strike may be the only way to have their demands heard (46). Nurses have watched as membership in the Union of American Physicians and the American Federation of Dentists and Physicians has grown. Physician members are mostly residents, interns, and the institutionally employed (47). Many allied health workers are now represented by major labor unions. In view of this, many nurses feel that they, too, should unionize.

Collective bargaining can be a two-edged sword. It can serve to promote the welfare of health care workers and begin to correct some of the problems which have plagued them—lack of career mobility, exploitation of students, and lack of day care and health care for employees. Unions can serve to promote better client care standards by addressing social concerns beyond the bread-and-butter issues of their members. They can promote the growth and development of the professions and enhance opportunities for career advancement for allied health workers. Conversely, unions can become so entrenched in wage and power issues that control of client care can slip from the hands of the professionals into those of union leaders and nonmedical administrators.

One method of avoiding these pitfalls of collective bargaining is for nurses to ask their own professional organization, the American Nurses Association, to represent them. Labor organizations, which were formed to serve other groups, often solicit nurse membership simply to boost their membership rolls, thus giving them more power to lobby with legislators, and not necessarily for the good of nursing or nurses (48). Whatever happens, collective bargaining has continued to play an important role in the evolution of health care delivery over the decade of the 1980s. What role it will play in the 1990s remains mere speculation in the face of health care reform.

Movements toward Change

It has always been safer to perpetuate a system than to change it. So it has seemed with our system of health care delivery over the past few decades. There are some cracks in the walls of the AMA-AHA-"Blues" dominated bastion, however. The '70s and '80s saw the emergence of a number of organizations and grassroots efforts that have directed part or all of their energies toward improving health care delivery. Among these are the Student Health Organization, the Medical Committee for Human Rights, the Women's Liberation Movement, and the Civil Rights Movement. No one solution will be a panacea for all the ills afflicting the health care delivery system and its impact on its providers. But, to paraphrase the Ehrenreichs, as the health care delivery system emerges, the differences between provider and consumer, between professional and allied health worker begin to blur. "No one is making it, and everyone has a stake in the creation of a revolutionary, people-oriented health system" (51).

References

1.   Bullough, B., and Bullough, V.L. (1972). Poverty, Ethnic Identity, and Health Care. New York: Appleton-Century-Crofts, pp. 157-168.
2.   Duffy, J. (1976). The Healers. New York: McGraw-Hill. p. 65.
3.   Health and Medical Services. (January, 1993). U.S. Industrial Outlook 1993. U.S. Department of Commerce.
4.   Statistical Abstract of the United States. 112th ed. (1992). Washington, DC: U.S. Department of Commerce, Bureau of the Census.
5.   Salaries of health care workers are healthy. (1993). Health Care Professional 3(3):6.
6.   Medical schools in the United States. (1982). Journal of the American Medical Association 248:3300-3317.
7.   McNutt, D.R. (1981). GMENAC: Its manpower forecasting framework. American Journal of Public Health 71(10):1116-1124.
8.   Budget breathes life into ailing children's prevention programs. (1993). The Nation's Health 23(5):1, 17-18.
9.   Geiger, H.J. (1993). Why don't medical students choose primary care? American Journal of Public Health 83:315-316.
10. Dolan, J. (1975). Three schools—1873. American Journal of Nursing 75(6):989-992.
11. Fact Sheet. (1989). Kansas City, MO: American Nurses Association.
12. Training the Nation's Health Manpower. (1972). Washington, DC: U.S. Department of Health, Education, and Welfare, Public Health Service.
13. Grupenhoff, J.T. and Strickland, S.P., eds. (1972). Federal Laws: Health Environment Manpower. Washington, DC: Science and Health Communications Group, pp. 1-7.
14. Report shows what it means to health to be disadvantaged. (1987). The Nation's Health 17(5,6):1-20.
15. Medical schools graduate fewer students in 1987. (1987). Chronicle of Higher Education 34(9):A2, A3.
16. Minorities and Women in the Health Fields. (1984). Washington, DC: U.S. Department of Health and Human Services, Public Health Service, Health Resources and Services Administration, Bureau of Health Professions.
17. Women's wages: The 59-cent solution. Editorial. (Feb. 17, 1980). The Boston Sunday Globe, p. G6.
18. Bennett, S.L. (1988). Comparable worth. Nursing and Health Care

9(5):245-247.

19. Dock, L.L. and Stewart, I.M. (1946). A Short History of Nursing, 4th ed. New York: G.P. Putnam's Sons, p. 254.

20. Ashley, J. (1976). Hospitals, Paternalism, and the Role of the Nurse. New York: Teachers College Press.

21. Goldmark, J. (1923). Nursing and Nursing Education in the United States: A Report of the Committee for the Study of Nursing Education. New York: Macmillan.

22. Ehrenreich, B. and English, D. (1973). Witches, Midwives and Nurses. Old Westbury, NY: Feminist Press, p. 30.

23. Kalisch, B.J. and Kalisch, P.A. (1976). The Cadet Nurse Corps in World War II. American Journal of Nursing 76(2):240-242.

24. Toward Quality of Nursing. Needs and Goals. (1963). Report of the Surgeon General's Consultant Group on Nursing. Washington, DC: U.S. Department of Health, Education, and Welfare, Public Health Service.

25. Rosenfeld, P. and Moses, E.B. (1988). Nursing supply and demand: An analysis of newspapers, journals and newsletters. Nursing and Health Care 9(5):249-252.

26. Nursing: A Social Policy Statement. (1980). Kansas City, MO: American Nurses Association.

27. The Scope of Nursing Practice. (1987). Kansas City, MO: American Nurses Association.

28. Unpublished report on nursing education and the supply of nurses. (1988). American Nurses Association.

29. American Nurses Association. (1988). Peer review guidelines. Kansas City, MO: American Nurses Association.

30. American Nurses Association. (1991). Standards of Clinical Nursing Practice. Kansas City, MO: American Nurses Association.

31. American Nurses Association. (1991). Standards for Nursing Staff Development. Kansas City, MO. American Nurses Association.

32. Practice of medicine is undergoing change, demoralizing doctors. (Feb. 18, 1990). The New York Times 1, 34-35.

33. Code for Nurses with Interpretive Statements. (1985). Kansas City, MO: American Nurses Association.

35. Lieb, R. (1978). Power, powerlessness and potential—nurse's role within the health care delivery system. Image 10(3):75-83.

36. Nursing wins JCAHO seat. (1992). The American Nurse 24(5):1.

37. While physician extenders proliferate, doctors worry about competition, care. (Aug. 5, 1992). Wall Street Journal, B1, B3.

38. Reverby, S. (1987). A caring dilemma: Womanhood and nursing in historical perspective. Nursing Research 36(1):5-11.

39. Brunt, B. (1992). Unlicensed assistive personnel. An education model for nursing. Council Perspective 1(3):1, 3.

40. Blegen, M.A., Gardner, D.L. and McCloskey, J.C. (1992). Who helps you with your work? American Journal of Nursing 93:26-31.

41. Kalisch, B.J. (1975). Of halfgods and mortals: Aesculapian authority. Nursing Outlook 23(1):22-28.

42. Leininger, M. (1976). Conflict and conflict resolutions. Theories and processes relevant to the health profession. In: M. Leininger, ed. Transcultural Health Care Issues and Conditions: Health Care Dimensions. Philadelphia: F.A. Davis, pp. 165-166.

43. Weiler, P.G. (1975). Health manpower dialectic—physician, nurse, physician assistant. American Journal of Public Health 65(8):858-863.

44. Zimmerman, A. (1975). Taft-Hartley amended. Implications for nursing. American Journal of Nursing 75(2):284-288.

45. Bloom, B.I. (1977). Collective action by professionals poses problems for administrations. Hospitals 51(6):167.

46. Miller, M.H. (1975). Nurses' right to strike. Journal of Nursing Administration 5(2):35.

47. Daniels, N. (1978). On the picket line. Are doctors' strikes ethical? Hastings Center Report 8(1):24.

48. Cleland, V. (1975). The professional model. American Journal of Nursing 75(2):288-292.

49. Young, Q.D. (1979). Unionization is major development in health. The Nation's Health 9(1):6.

50. Safriet, B.J. (1992). Health care dollars and regulatory sense: The role of advanced practice nursing. Yale Journal on Regulation 9:417-488.

51. Ehrenreich, J. and Ehrenreich, B. (1976). Hospital workers: A case study in the "new working class." In D. Kotelchuck, ed., Prognosis Negative. New York: Vintage Books, p. 241.

52. Secretary's Commission on Nursing Final Report. (1988). Washington, DC: Department of Health and Human Services.

53. The National Health Service Corps. (1992). Summary Fact Sheet.

54. National League for Nursing. (1992). Nursing School Applications, enrollments, and graduations. New York: NLN.

55. Ellis, J.R. and Hartley, C.L. (1992). Nursing in Today's World. 4th ed. Philadelphia: Lippincott.

56. Federal regulations to prevent infection of health-care workers will be costly. (July 2, 1992). Wall Street Journal, B1, 5.

57. Mikulencak, M. (1992). Personal safety emerging as chief workplace concern. The American Nurse 24(10):1, 7.

58. Kohler, S. (1992). Workload, low salaries create RN job stress. The American Nurse 24(10):2.

59. Enrollment of nursing students is up, nursing vacancy rates are down in 1990s. (1993). The Nation's Health 23(2):4.

7

Inadequacies in the Health Care Delivery System

"In the United States poor people are sicker than non-poor people, blacks and chicanos are sicker than whites, and rural people are sicker than urban people. The sicker groups generally get less medical care" (1, p. 10).

The health care delivery system, as we know it in the United States, does not meet the needs of all the citizens. There are those who are either ignored or exploited by the system, and those who encounter barriers even when attempts are made to reach them. Lack of information, inability to pay, maldistribution of providers and services, transportation difficulties, inconvenient clinic hours, language problems, and attitudes of caretakers are some of the barriers encountered by those who fall between the cracks. Devoid of political clout, these people are also ill equipped to bring about any change in the system.

In selecting a sample of underserved groups for presentation here, it became apparent immediately that poverty affects many or all of these groups. For that reason, issues of health care for the poor will be addressed first and then the discussion will center on several other groups that our present system has either ignored, exploited, or failed to serve adequately. The intent of this chapter is to provide some of the tools needed to assess a selected population and identify the barriers to health care that confront it.

The Poor

"The poor in the United States receive a disproportionately low share of health services" (2). By 1990, it was estimated that nearly 12.6 million children live in poverty. In 1990, nearly one million persons lost their health insurance (16). Between 1989 and 1991, 4.2 million persons were added to the ranks of the poor; 44% were African-American and Hispanic (21). Medicare and Medicaid have failed to close the gap, indicating that money alone is not the solution. The poor are often elderly, children, women, and/or members of ethnic or racial minorities. The use of health care services by the poor is sporadic and often inappropriate, crisis oriented, episodic, symptomatic, impersonal, and uncoordinated. To treat peoples' illnesses and send them back to environments where they are cold and hungry most of the time is as futile as plugging a hole in a dam with chewing gum. Band-Aid attempts at health care do not encourage utilization nor do they address prevention.

The poor have shorter life expectancies, higher infant morbidity and mortality rates, and greater physical limitations resulting from chronic disease; further, they continue to suffer from diseases which have been virtually eradicated from the upper economic stratum of the population. (4, 77).

Often without health insurance, unable to qualify for Medicaid (23) or, even if insured, unable to pay for deductibles or co-payments, the poor are wedged into a fragmented system. Preventive care, e.g., immunization and screening, is often obtained in settings that focus on wellness not covered by insurance and not accepting Medicaid clients. Thus, since health insurance in this country is, by and large, illness insurance, the poor are less likely to be able to afford to keep well.

Illness care is sought through private physicians, clinics, or, in many cases, emergency rooms. The necessity of paying fees prior to or upon receipt of service renders many of these services inaccessible. Lack of transportation or lack of babysitters are other barriers. Clinic hours often mean that a client loses a day of work, a hardship for those paid by the hour or for piecework. Impersonal, assembly-line care means having to give your history over and over each time you go for care. Illiteracy or speaking only a language other than English means inability to fill out forms and understand directions for diet, medication, and other modes of therapy. This frequently results in the client being branded as "noncompliant" or "uncooperative." Public clinics are often located in large medical centers where one may be relegated to the unenviable position of "guinea pig" for a host of medical students, interns, and residents who may never see the same patient twice (5,p.11). The attitudes of providers, who are usually white and middle-class, may interfere with the process of health care delivery.

Environmental factors impact on health in important ways. The poor may lack heat and sanitary facilities and may experience inadequate diets, vermin and parasites, occupational hazards, long hours for low pay, and the psychological stresses of chronic poverty (6). The effects of these are seen in more frequent and longer-lasting illnesses. In the 1990s, the homeless have been added to those who suffer the effects of environment and lack of access to care.

By the beginning of the 1990s, homeless persons as a subset of those living in poverty in the United State numbered anywhere from one-half million to three million. Of these, approximately 35% are families with children. The health care needs and problems of homeless persons are more severe than those of poor persons with a permanent residence. The problems of access to care experienced by persons living in poverty are exacerbated by homelessness. Lack of a permanent address and/or a job can limit access to even the publicly funded programs. Since many homeless shelters do not allow their residents to stay during daytime hours, taking medications, following self-care recommendations, and keeping appointments become problems with many dimensions (17).

Solutions

A number of model programs have been established in attempts to overcome the barriers for the poor and to provide access to the health care system for them. The findings of some experiments in health care provision to homeless persons, to those eligible for Medicaid, and for pregnant women emphasize the importance of addressing the priorities of clients (7,16,17,18,20). Including the target population in policy making, planning, and implementing neighborhood health programs has a significant impact on their utilization (8). Programs such as the Erie Family Health Center that provide health care of, by, and for the poor, and are nursing managed, demonstrate the value that the poor place on health services (9). (See Chapter 4.)

Most important to any attempt to remove barriers are·l) an understanding of the environments of poverty and 2) the ability to plan programs that not only provide health care but that also alter those factors which render that care only marginally beneficial. Until we can find ways to wage a more effective war on poverty, our efforts to improve health care delivery will be thwarted. Expansion of Medicaid benefits to working families above the federal poverty level, legislation in several states for health care for everyone, and demonstration projects with Medicaid clients in HMOs are important attempts to better understand and make a significant impact upon the interactions between social conditions and health (16).

Minorities

All too often, our poor are members of groups that have been discriminated against by our health care system. African-Americans, those of Hispanic descent, Native Americans, and Asian-Americans suffer not only lack of access to adequate health care but a significantly lop-sided representation in the subsystem of providers. They are disproportionately represented in unskilled jobs within the health care system and minimally present as professionals. Implications for interactions between clients and caregivers are important and obvious (5,pp. 147-157).

Blatant discrimination in the form of denying health care to individuals on the basis of race is one of the saddest sagas in all our history. Ironically, it is the power of the dollar that has been most influential in decreasing such discrimination since, in order to qualify for Medicare and Medicaid reimbursement, individual providers and institutions have had to abandon practices which could be interpreted as discriminatory. Thus, discriminatory practices were often discontinued, not out of a belief in equality, but in order to qualify for federal health care dollars (5, pp. 157-162).

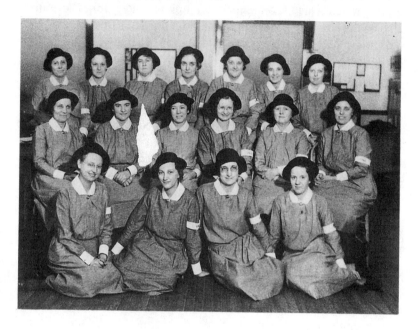

Fig. 7.1. Chicago Visiting Nurse Association, 1926.

That we have not yet achieved equality and freedom from discrimination in care is evidenced in data from a number of studies. Statistics showing life expectancies and high infant mortality rates among non-whites bear witness to inequalities within our society (4,77,78). To bring about equal access to quality health care for all will not eliminate the effects of poverty on the quality and length of life. To continue to use poverty as an excuse to deny access, however, deprives a substantial number of Americans of what many have come to believe is a basic human right.

Solutions

Programs to encourage the recruitment of members of minority groups into health professions are increasing in number and success (5). Such efforts are exemplified by the work of the minority task force of the National Student Nurse Association, which assists disadvantaged students who would otherwise be shut out of a profession.

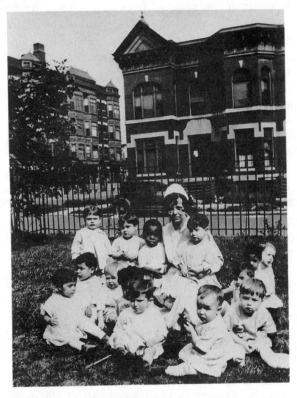

Fig. 7.2. One of the Visiting Nurses who worked out of Hull House Station in Chicago in the 1920s on duty at the Children's Home.

Recognition of the impact of race on health care delivery is reflected in books that address issues of race and culture as they relate to nursing care (10,11). The founding of the Council on Cultural

Diversity in Nursing is evidence of increasing awareness on the part of nurses, as health care providers, of the importance of recognizing and assessing the impact of cultural factors on health and illness care (12). These are important beginnings to full integration of minorities into the health care delivery system, both as providers and as consumers. This is not to suggest that persons of diverse ethnic and racial backgrounds be asked to divest themselves of their heritage and openly embrace "the system," but rather that health professionals be made aware of their problems and of how best to collaborate with them in the interest of better health care for all of our citizens.

Important federal initiatives to address health care issues for persons from diverse ethnic backgrounds occurred with the establishment of the Office of Minority Health in 1985 and initiatives through that office (30).

Rural Americans

Citizens of the rural areas of our country continue to have more unmet health care needs and fewer health care resources than urban residents (3). There are as many barriers to access for these people as there are special conditions that impact on health and health care.

Geography is one of the most ubiquitous barriers to access to health care. In some large western states particularly, distances are great and population sparse. The U.S. Census of Population defines "rural" people as those who live in a place with fewer than 2,500 persons or in the open countryside. While it is true that some of our wealthiest citizens live in areas that can be characterized as rural, a disproportionate number of rural Americans are poor and elderly, have low educational attainments, and live in substandard housing (3).

Several of the critical issues that affect rural health care are: a higher proportion of residents who live below the federal poverty level than in urban or suburban areas; a predominance of two-parent families, thus ruling out those families' eligibility for Medicaid; substandard housing; impure water and inadequate sanitation facilities; fewer hospital beds per capita; fewer nursing homes and other facilities for the elderly; lower federal expenditures for health care than for urban residents; and fewer professional health care providers (doctors, dentists, nurses, and so on) per capita (73).

High infant mortality rates, a significantly higher occurrence of chronic, treatable health conditions, dental problems, mental illness, and malnutrition are other important health problems for rural Americans (3). Occupational risks for health are also great; they include exposure to dangerous machinery and pesticides. Location in relation to urban centers, climate,geography,poverty, lack of medical insurance, and maldistribution of providers and services may all have a part in the lack of adequate services to rural people. Further, with hospitals experiencing declining censuses, many rural hospitals have been forced to close, making care less accessible. Rural hospitals are more likely to be state or local government owned, less likely to have resident programs or to be part of a multi-hospital system, and unlikely to offer any services beyond the routine (13,pp.8-9; 14).

Solutions

A number of important programs have been initiated since the passing of the Hill-Burton Act (National Hospital Survey and Construction Act) in 1946. This act prompted a large increase in the quantity and quality of hospital facilities in rural areas (16). Unfortunately, it did little to alter the maldistribution of persons to staff those hospitals.

Some of the efforts to improve health care delivery to rural clients and to help overcome problems of maldistribution and mobility of caregivers in the target rural population are in the form of demonstration projects (15). Revitalization of the National Health Service Corps has also helped to bring health care professionals to rural areas. So has the establishment of community health centers in rural areas.

Significant legislation passed in 1977—Public Law 95-210 (the Rural Health Services Clinic Act)—allows for the establishment, under federal guidelines, of rural health clinic services and reimbursement of nurse practitioners and physician assistants by Medicare and Medicaid. This reimbursement may occur for services not directly supervised by a physician, an important point when one considers the paucity of physicians in some of our rural areas (24). Nurses working in expanded and extended roles in collaboration with physicians and/or as primary health care providers are important to the improvement of rural health care (31,33).

Migrant Farm Workers

The number of migrant farm workers in this country is over five million, 85% of them minorities (34). The problems of the migrant are significant and mirror those of rural Americans. In addition, migrant families face problems in relation to health and health care that are unique to their migratory status.

Woody Guthrie immortalized migrant farmers in his famous song, "Pastures of Plenty" (28). Images of the stream of migrant workers moving north with the crops, living in shacks with no sanitary facilities, and endlessly enslaved by the bosses and the company store persist in spite of the unionization of some workers and improved working conditions. Issues of survival and humane conditions and wages are now accompanied by demands for a decrease in the use of pesticides, research on the safety of chemicals, and employee benefit packages.

Robert Coles, a psychiatrist who has spent a great deal of time being with and studying migrant families, quoted one migrant woman as saying, "My children, they suffer, I know. They hurts and I can't stop it. I just have to pray that they'll stay alive somehow" (29).

Migrant farm workers are defined as persons who for long periods of time must move far from the place they call home to work in the fields of others. The "California stream," as those from the California area are called, is the largest group, and its members are mostly Mexican-Americans although some are Anglos. Then there is the "Texas" or "midcontinent stream," comprised mostly of Mexican-Americans and some Native Americans, and the Florida-based "eastern stream," consisting mostly of African-Americans plus some Puerto Ricans, Jamaicans, Haitians, Mexican-Americans, and Anglos.

Migrant families tend to be large. Half of the workers are less than 25 years of age, with an equal number of men and women. Children also go to work in the fields, often illegally. The mean family income is $5,921, $4,638 coming from farm work, with work days averaging less than half the year. Forty-eight percent have less schooling than the ninth grade. Housing is generally substandard. The average life expectancy is only 49 years. (41)

The health problems of migrants include tuberculosis and other infectious diseases, parasite infestation, chronic diseases, nerve and back injuries, pesticide poisoning, malnutrition, dental problems, multiple pregnancies, uncorrected congenital deformities, and gunshot wounds. These conditions result in a high mortality rate for infants and high morbidity and mortality rates for all others (32, 42).

Contributory factors and barriers include lack of access to care, detrimental environments, occupational hazards, mobility, ineligibility for Medicare and Medicaid, lack of health insurance, inability to speak English, superstition, fear, limited education, and lack of facilities for care. In addition, many migrants are illegal aliens, making them fearful of and/or ineligible for health care even where it exists (14,p.34).

Solutions

Several demonstration projects and pieces of legislation represent attempts to provide more adequate care for migrant workers. Organizations of farm workers, the Migrant Legal Action program in particular, have prevailed upon OSHA to set fairly good standards for the use of pesticides and some regulations regarding the safe use of farm equipment. Monies for public health programs have become available through the Department of Health and Human Services (34). Twenty years ago, the United Farm Workers AFL/CIO in California negotiated contracts with provisions for health insurance, health care, and housing, and the union began to sponsor clinics (37, p.845). Recent changes in Medicaid regulations make more seasonal agricultural families eligible (35). In 1988, the long-awaited Department of Labor ruling on sanitation for migrant worker housing was finally issued and funds were increased dramatically for migrant health centers (36, 42). The migrant health branch of the Division of Primary

Care Services of the U.S. Department of Health and Human Services oversees migrant health. The Migrant Clinicians Network, including many nurses, has worked on a plan for migrant health care (43).

Native Americans and Alaska Natives

Native Americans and Alaska Natives are among our most rural and most impoverished citizens (26). According to some sources, there are about one million Native Americans and Alaska Natives in well over 500 federally recognized tribes scattered throughout our 50 states (5, p. 89). Another source cites more than 250 federally recognized tribes—some 1,420,000 Native Americans and Alaskan Natives. Many of these people live on reservations in 25 states, the majority of which are in the western half of the country. Tribal lands exceed 41,000,000 acres (73).

Alaska has over 76,000 Eskimos, Aleuts, Athebaskan, Tsimpsian, Tlingit, and Haida peoples scattered over 33,000 miles of coastline and along the rivers in villages of 30 to 1,000 people. There are no tribal organizations as there are in the contiguous 48 states (39). These Americans are subject to all the problems of access to health care that plague our rural population. In addition, strong healing traditions may be in conflict with or disregarded by the white provider. Many Native Americans still reside on reservations, often in inadequate housing with scant sanitary facilities. Unemployment is high, and employment is often seasonal and hazardous—fighting forest fires, for example.

Common problems include tuberculosis, a high infant and maternal mortality rate, otitis media, diabetes, alcoholism, malnutrition, lower life expectancy, fatal accidents, and suicide (72).

Caught in a conflict between tradition and twentieth-century American culture, Native Americans and Alaska Natives are subject to stresses which affect their mental health. Their children frequently display emotional problems and behavior disorders (38, p.9).

Barriers to care include isolation on reservations, a lack of providers, poverty, lack of articulation between tribal healers and Anglo providers, low educational level, and lack of transportation (reservations may extend hundreds of miles).

Solutions

Since 1955, when the Indian Health Service came under the aegis of the Department of Health, Education, and Welfare, significant changes have occurred for the better in provision of health care (40). In 1976, Public Law 94-437 was passed expanding Indian health services. It includes provisions for increasing the number of Native Americans and Alaska Natives in the health professions to provide services to their people. It also provides for upgrading health facilities, for new construction, for outreach programs, and for health services for urban Native Americans (44). The Indian Self-Determination Assistance Act (P.L. 93-638) provides Indians with an opportunity to control their own programs and has been amended to expand this control (76).

The Indian Health Service operates 43 general hospitals, 66 health centers, 60 health stations, and 5 school health stations. Tribes and urban groups manage and operate 364 health care facilities to serve Native Americans and Alaska Natives (46). The Alaska Area Native Health Service, part of the Indian Health Service, serves the native residents of our largest state with 7 hospitals, 4 Indian Health Service Area Offices, 8 health centers, 7 health stations, and 130 village clinics (39). Under the Older Americans Act Amendments of 1987, an office for Native American Programs was created to oversee and administer services to Native American older adults (40). Over 2,400 nurses serve in the Indian Health Service and have developed innovative programs for care delivery (47,48).

Prisoners

In several thousand federal, state, county, and local prisons and jails across the United States there are, on any given day, a million inmates (45), half of whom are serving sentences and half of whom are awaiting conviction or release. Close to three million persons are under correctional supervision each year. Most prisoners are poor and young, and African-American and other minorities are vastly over-represented. The number of women prisoners is increasing, although women have always been a minority in prisons. Women now constitute 4.9% of prisoners, a 15.1% increase in 10 years (56). More than a quarter of our prisoners are in prisons constructed 70 or more years ago.

The health problems of prisoners include mental disorders, drug and alcohol abuse, chronic diseases characteristic of the general population, lymphadenopathy, viral hepatitis, foreign body in gastroin-testinal tract, dental caries, pulmonary tuberculosis, AIDS, and injury from prison jobs or peers. There is a lack of health care facilities, and personnel problems are severe. Most prisons are located in remote areas, the work they offer employees is routine, and health worker contacts with prisoners can usually only be made when guards are in attendance. Organizational constraints include a high priority for security, a low priority for personnel, a low budget for health care, a lack of leadership, a lack of facilities for care, and the dangers involved when drugs are moved and when nurses and doctors must go in and out of cells and cell areas (75). Prisoners may abuse or "con" the system to get out of work, to get a chance to escape, or to obtain drugs, which are prison "currency" (69).

During the 1970s, a number of exposés of prison conditions incited public interest (49,50,5l). In l988, a Supreme Court ruling upheld prisoners' rights to health care (74). In 1990, with burgeoning prison populations, new concerns have arisen about the health of prisoners and the notably increased prevalence of mental illness among them (45). An aging prison population also raises special concerns for health care (55). So do the health care needs of women prisoners (56).

Solutions

In 1974, the American Nurses Association passed a resolution on health care in correctional institutions (52). In 1976, the American Public Health Association issued a formal list of standards for health services in correctional institutions (53). In 1977, the American Medical Association investigated prison health and as a result launched a drive to improve medical care for prisoners. That organization has also drafted codes of minimum standards for such care (54).

Changes in health care by the New York City Prison Health Service represent an attempt to implement these resolutions and standards (52). A pilot project in Chicago utilizes former medical corpsmen to expand services for inmates (58). The use of a comprehensive data collection system in New York State facilities will help to provide documentation of needs and resources (59). Encouraging prospects for change are evident in pilot projects on prison health including nurse practitioner care in an HMO model (56,70).

Older Adults

As the population of the United States ages, the health care needs of older adults become more apparent and more critical. Unpaid caregivers for seniors are usually women, and often they are elderly and frail themselves (57). By 2020, it is projected that there will be more than 50 million older adults in the U.S., 10 million of whom will be at home but in need of care (65, 83). For those who do require long-term care, and for whom care at home is not an option, paying for care will pose an immense burden on individuals, their families, and society as a whole. Although poverty rates for older adults have fallen over the past decade, they have not done so for women: 15.2% of women 65 and over (2.5 million) live below the federal poverty level as opposed to 8.5% of men. For women 85 and older, the rate is l9.7% (71). This has important implications for access to health care. Given the likelihood that an older person will have one or more chronic diseases, and the increasing rate of disability the older one becomes, health care needs emerge as a major issue.

Solutions

Advocacy groups for older Americans have become increasingly vocal over the past two decades. Their ability to assert influence on policy makers is critical to social change needed at the legislative level to assure care for our aging population. Examining health policy as it evolves for its implications for the aging population is important. Of course, health policy should not be disconnected from social policy as it affects seniors (79). Nurses often serve as advocates for their patients by demanding justice for all (80). Innovative programs developed by nurses for older adults help them remain as independent as possible for as long as possible (82).

Women

When considering social resources, and those include health care regardless of income, place of residence, ethnic or social background, women are discriminated against (60). More frequently than men, women interact with the health care system both as consumers (in part due to childbearing), and also because they bear the major responsibility for the health of family members (61).

The Victorian era contributed in its own unique way to the oppression of women and the perpetuation of age-old myths of inferiority and frailty. Not only were such accoutrements of the age as tight corsets hazardous to health, but, in addition, women were prevented from getting exercise by the misguided belief in feminine frailty. Of course, women were exposed to the risks of pregnancy and childbirth, but the basic reason for the debilitation of upper and middle-class women was the product of a vicious circle of weakness, lack of exercise, and a sedentary life.

Interestingly, economics played a critical role in the mythology of the times surrounding women's health. Since poor women could not afford health care, physicians were not particularly interested in them as clients. Likewise, since they posed little threat to the profession as potential members, lacking as they were in even basic education, little heed was paid to perpetuating the myth of feminine frailty among this group.

Essential to the very survival of the poor family was the income brought in by female as well as male household members. Consequently, poor women worked long hours at tedious, repetitive, and often hazardous tasks in mills, factories, and sweatshops, or did household tasks at a pittance for the frail sisters of the upper classes. Obvious as it may seem, the incongruity of the medical philosophy and the deprivations suffered by a large proportion of half the human race passed almost unnoticed.

Suffice it to say, provisions of health care for all the maladies attributed to the wealthier classes filled the purse of many a physician. One need only read nineteenth-century medical texts to find extensive accounts of the maladies and the treatments prescribed, all designed to produce maximum dependency of patient upon provider and thus perpetuate yet another myth.

For the doctors, the myth of female frailty served two purposes. It helped them to disqualify women as healers, and of course, it made women highly qualified as patients (62).

Woman's role as consumer of health care has enlarged over the past century. Not only do women form a disproportionate client caste for health care, but they have often suffered humiliation at the hands of health care providers. For example, pharmaceutical ads in medical journals depict women in ways that are stereotyped and demeaning (63).

Evidence is accumulating that blatant overprescription of tranquilizers for women is common practice. Estrogens, notably DES, continue to be used without adequate warnings to consumers. Our most effective contraceptive method, the pill, is unquestionably dangerous for some women. Women take 50% more prescription drugs than men (66). Health insurance for women is often tied to that of their husbands. The rates of surgical procedures such as hysterectomies, cesarean sections, and even radical mastectomies are high (65). Issues of women as research subjects that are reminiscent of the DES scandal are present in the current tomoxifen study.

More women are poor, and since women are more likely to work part time they are less likely to have the health insurance they need, especially if they are heads of households (64). Insurance coverage for childbearing is inadequate and for contraception nonexistent except in HMOs (67). Around 1990, the exclusion of women in research studies exploded in the news (68). Suddenly women's health issues moved into the spotlight. The federal government created the Office of Research in Women's Health at NIH and mandated inclusion of women in study populations (22).

Solutions

The self-help and self-care movements, the close ties between the women's movement and health issues, and the alternatives to traditional care that are emerging are not accidents. In increasing numbers, women are protesting the insensitivity and exploitation they have been dealt by the health delivery system. The deluge of lay literature on health and body issues attests to this interest. Women's self-help health clinics have sprung up coast to coast, offering alternative models of care for and by women.

The dramatic numbers of women and their partners enrolling in childbirth education classes, and the incredible changes in medical practices in labor and delivery, reflect the pressures of consumers for more control and a stronger voice in the important experience of giving birth. Birth centers, home births, and birthing rooms all exist primarily because of consumer demands.

Within the government, women's councils have begun to emerge to provide advice on policy, programs, and legislation. In any move toward a national health service or national health insurance as we grapple with health care reform, much attention must be focused on righting the discrimination and inequalities involved in health care for women.

The future is bright if women will implement change by using the power that is theirs by virtue of their numbers. The appointment of women to more cabinet posts and administrative positions within government is one positive sign of progress.

References

1. Shenkin, B.N. (1974). Health Care for Migrant Workers: Policies and Politics. Cambridge, MA: Ballinger.
2. Bergner, L. and Yerby, A.S. (1976). Low incomes and barriers to use of health services. In: R.L. Kane, J.M. Kasteler, and R.M. Gray, eds. The Health Gap: Medical Services and the Poor. New York: Springer, p. 37.
3. Reed, S. and Sautler, R.C. (1990). Children of Poverty. Kappan Special Report.
4. Wilkinson, R.G. (1992). National mortality rates: The impact of inequality. American Journal of Public Health 82(8):1082-1084.
5. Bullough, B. and Bullough, V.L. (1982). Health Care for the Other Americans. East Norwalk, CT: Appleton-Century-Crofts.
6. Kosa, J. (1969). The nature of poverty. In: J. Kosa, A. Antonovsky, and I.K. Zola, eds., Poverty and Health: A Sociological Analysis. Cambridge, MA: Harvard University Press, pp. 21-25.
7. Robertson, M.J. and Cousineau, M.R. (1986). Health status and access to health services among the urban homeless. American Journal of Public Health 76(5):561-563.
8. Kane, T.J. (1987). Giving back control: Long-term poverty and motivation. Social Service Review 61(3):405-419.
9. Lang, N.M. (1983). Nurse-managed centers. Will they thrive? American Journal of Nursing 83(9):1290-1296.
10. Leininger, M. (1991). Cultural Care Diversity and Universality: A Theory of Nursing. New York: National League for Nursing.
11. Spector, R. (1991). Cultural Diversity in Health and Illness. 3rd ed. East Norwalk, CT: Appleton-Lange.
12. Organizational Structure. (1984). Unpublished organization chart. American Nurses Association.
13. Urban and Rural Hospital Costs: 1981-1985. (1988). U.S. Department of Health and Human Services, National Center for Health Services Research and Health Care Technology Assessment.
14. McLaughlin, C.P., Ricketts, T.C., Freund, D.A., and Sheps, C.O. (1985). An evaluation of subsidized rural primary care programs. American Journal of Public Health 75(7):749-753.
15. Henderson, F.C. (1988). Non-competitive linkages: A collaboration model for family-centered adolescent health promotion. In: Proceedings of the Fifth Annual Nursing Research Conference, Pace University,

New York.

16. Liu, J.T., Regan, C., Orloff, T.M. and Rivera, L.A (1992). The Health of America's Children. Washington, DC: Children's Defense Fund.

17. Wagner, J.D. and Menke, E.M. (1992). Case management of homeless families. Clinical Nurse Specialist 6(2):65-71.

18. Berne, A.S., Dato, C., Mason, D.J. and Rafferty, M. (1990). A nursing model for addressing the health needs of homeless families. Image 22(1):8-13.

19. Moscovice, I.S. and Rosenblatt, R.A. (1982). Rural health care delivery amidst federal retrenchment. American Journal of Public Health 72(12):1380-1385.

20. Mastragelo, R. (1993). House of hospitality. Advance for Nurse Practitioners 1(2):9,18,20.

21. Numbers of uninsured continue growing, says group. (1992). The Nation's Health 22(2):8.

22. The Society for the Advancement of Women's Health Research. (1991). Towards a Women's Health Research Agenda: Findings of the Scientific Advisory Meeting.

23. Stevens, P.E. (1993). Who gets care? Access to health care as an arena for nursing action. In: B.K.-M, ed. Who Gets Health Care? New York: Springer, pp. 13-26.

24. Rural Clinics Act offers revenue benefits. (1988). The Nurse Practitioner 13(8):64-66.

25. Abrams, R. (1987). HMOs end Medicaid: Issues and prospects. Studies and Papers, Vol. V, pp. 1-7. Rockville, MD: Health Resources and Services Administration.

26. Health Status of Minorities and Low-Income Groups. (1985). U.S. Department of Health and Human Services, Public Health Service, Health Resources and Services, Bureau of Health Professions, Division of Disadvantaged Assistance.

27. The National Health Service Corps. (1992). Summary Fact Sheet:1-3.

28. Guthrie, W.W. (1960). Pastures of Plenty. New York: Ludlow Music, Inc.

29. Coles, R. (1967). Migrants, sharecroppers, mountaineers. Children of Crisis, Vol. II. Boston: Little, Brown, p. 62.

30. Toward Equality of Well-Being: Strategies for Improving Minority Health. (1993). Washington, DC: Office of Minority Health, U.S. Department of Health and Human Services.

31. Wasem, C. (1990). The Rural Health Clinics Services Act: A sleeping

giant of reimbursement. Journal of the American Academy of Nurse Practitioners 2(2):85-87.

32. Arbab, D.M. and Weidner, B.L. (1986). Infectious diseases and field water supply and sanitation among migrant farm workers. American Journal of Public Health 76(6):694-695.

33. Bigbee, J.L. (1992). Frontier areas: Opportunities for NPs' primary care services. The Nurse Practitioner 17(9):47-48, 50, 53-54, 57.

34. Migrant Health. (1990). Rockville, MD: National Migrant Resource Program.

35. Legalized eligibility for key federal assistance programs. (1987). Child Health Financing Report 5:1,3.

36. Senate boosts funds for migrant and community health center. (1988). The Nation's Health 18(7):5.

37. Moses, M. (1973). "Viva la Causa!" American Journal of Nursing 73(5):842-848.

38. Indian Health Service. (1986). The Indian Health Program. Washington, D.C.: U.S. Department of Health and Human Service, Public Health Service, Health Resources and Services Administration.

39. Nursing Assignment: Alaska Service Area. (1991). Washington, DC: Indian Health Service.

40. OAA amendments call for new federal office on Indian aging. (1988). NIBH Health Reporter 4(8):14-15.

41. An Atlas of State Profiles Which Estimate Number of Migrant and Seasonal Farm Workers and Members of Their Families. (1990). Rockville, MD: Migrant Health Branch, U.S. Department of Health and Human Services.

42. Migrant and Seasonal Farm Worker Health Objectives for the Year 2000. (1990). Rockville, MD: National Migrant Resource Program.

43. Blueprint for Migrant Health: Health Care Delivery to the Year 2000. (1992). Rockville, MD: Migrant Clinicians Network Monograph Series.

44. Shenson, D., Dubler, N., and Michaels, D. (1990). Jails and prisons: The new asylums? American Journal of Public Health 80(6):655-656.

45. Mortiz, P. (1982) Health care in correctional facilities: A nursing challenge. Nursing Outlook 30(4):253-259.

46. Indian Health Service. (no date). Indian Health Service Hospitals and Area Offices. Rockville, MD: Indian Health Service.

47. McCarty, P. (1990). Indian health center fills community gap. The American Nurse 22(8):8,9.

48. McLaughlin, R. (1993): Houses, not tepees. Advance for Nurse

Practitioners 1(1):22.

49. Minton, R.J., ed. (1971). Inside Prison American Style. New York: Vintage.

50. Burkhart, K.W. (1976). Women in Prison. New York: Popular Library.

51. Wicker, T.A. (1975). A Time to Die. New York: Quadrangle.

52. Murtha, R. (1975). Change in one city's system. American Journal of Nursing 75(3):421-422.

53. Prison health standards. (1976). The Nation's Health 6(11):3.

54. Robinson, D. (1977). The scandalous medical care in our jails. Parade 10-12.

55. Colsher, P.L., Wallace, R.B., Loeffelholz, P.L. and Sales, M. (1992). Health status of older male prisoners: A comprehensive survey. American Journal of Public Health 82:881-884.

56. Wilson, J.S. and Leasure, R. (1991). Cruel and unusual punishment: The health care of women in prison. The Nurse Practitioner 16(2):32, 34,36,38,39.

57. Exploding the Myths: Caregiving in America. (1988). U.S. House of Representatives Select Committee on Aging.

58. King, L., Reynolds, A., and Young, Q. (1977). Utilization of former military medical corpsmen in the provision of jail health services. American Journal of Public Health 67(8):730-734.

59. Froom, J., Howe, B., Mangone, D., Swearingen, C. and Warren, P.S. (1977). A health data system for New York State correctional facilities. American Journal of Public Health 67(3):250-251.

60. Milio, N. (1975). The Care of Health in Communities: Access for Outcasts. New York: MacMillan, p. 35.

61. Wallen, J., Waitzkin, H., and Stoeckle, J.D. (1979). Physician stereotypes about female health and illness. Women and Health 4:135-146.

62. Ehrenreich, B. and English, D. Complaints and Disorders: The Sexual Politics of Sickness. Old Westbury, NY: The Feminist Press, p. 23.

63. Hawkins, J.W. and Aber, C.S. (1993). Women in advertisements in medical journals. Sex Roles 28(3/4):233-242.

64. Wilson, J.B. (1988). Women and poverty. Women and Health: 12(3/4):21-40.

65. Older Women's League. (1990). A Challenge for the 1990's: Improving Health or Women. Older Women's League.

66. Ogur, B. (1986). Long day's journal into night. Women and Health II(1):99-115.

67. Jallon, J.R. and Block, R. (1988). Changing patterns of health insur-

ance coverage. Women and Health 12(3/4):120-136.

68. Dresser, R. (1992). Wanted single white male for medical research. Hastings Center Report 22(1:24-29.

69. Chaisson, G.M. (1981). Correctional health care—beyond the barriers. American Journal of Nursing 81(4):737-738.

70. Little, L.A. (1981). Change process for prison health nursing. American Journal of Nursing 81(4):739-742.

71. Stone, R. (1989). The Feminization of Poverty Among the Elderly. Washington, DC: National Center for Health Services Research and Health Care Technology Assessment.

72. Indian Health Service. (1986). Rockville, MD: Indian Health Service.

73. Statistical Abstracts of the United States, 112th ed. (1992). Washington, DC: US Department of Commerce, Bureau of the Census.

74. Supreme Court ruling reinforces right to adequate health care in prisons. (1988). The Nation's Health 18(8):1,11.

75. Krupp, L.B., Gelberg, E.A., and Wormser, G.P. (1987). Prisoners as medical patients. American Journal of Public Health 77(7):859-860.

76. IHS expands PL 100-472 process to involve more tribal participants. (1989). NIHB Health Reporter 4(12):1,2.

77. Fingerhut, L.A. and Makuc, D.M. (1992). Mortality among minority populations in the United States. American Journal of Public Health 82(8):1168-1170.

78. Hispanic health and nutrition examination survey, 1982-84: Findings on health status and health care needs. (1990). American Journal of Public Health 80 (Dec. suppl.) whole issue.

79. Williamson, J.B., Shindal, J.A., and Evans, L. (1985). Aging and Public Policy. Springfield, IL: Charles Thomas.

80. Fleck, L.M. (1987). Decisions of justice and health care. Journal of Gerontological Nursing 13(3):40-46.

81. Jamieson, M. and Campbell, J. (1987). The St. Anthony Park block nurse program. American Journal of Public Health 77(9):1227-1228.

82. Hawkins, J.W., Utley, Q.E., Igou, J.F., and Johnson, E.E. (1991). Intradisciplinary nursing practice in a wellness center for older adults. Aging Network News 9(4):4,6.

83. Haunting issues for the U.S. Caring for the elderly ill. (1990, March 27). The New York Times 1, A18.

8

The Health Care Industry

The health care industry, privately owned and existing for profit, contributes substantially both to health care delivery and health care costs. The number of vendors relating to private providers and public institutions has mushroomed along with the expansion of health care delivery. One has only to scan the shelves of the local drug store or the utility room of a hospital unit to realize how many companies are in the business of supplying goods and services related to health care. Over 300 manufacturers belong to the Health Industry Manufacturers Association (25).

In addition, proprietary institutions and agencies offering health services have increased dramatically in number. Nursing homes, convalescent and long-term hospitals, home health care service agencies, freestanding ambulatory care (known as "doc in a box") and surgical centers, managed care groups including for-profit HMOs, medical equipment and supply stores, dialysis centers, drug store chains, freestanding medical laboratories, and agencies hawking professional and nonprofessional staff on a "Kelly Girl" basis are but a few examples.

Gone are the days when hospitals sterilized and reused most

supplies and did their own laundry, and when all providers except physicians and adjunct services personnel were employees of the institution. Some of the innovations, such as disposable gloves, needles, and syringes, have led to safer care, whereas others, it could be argued, have merely contributed to escalation of costs.

The Pharmaceutical Industry

Drugs have been used since the earliest recordings of history. In ancient times, people used roots, herbs, leaves, water, urine, earth, animal parts, and virtually all manner of natural materials for preventing and treating illnesses. When the first colonists arrived in North America, only a few dozen effective drugs were known, although there were literally hundreds of simple drugs and compounds listed in existing pharmacopoeia (1, p. 2). These included mercury, used as a purgative and later for the treatment of syphilis; ergot, used for preventing hemorrhage after childbirth; digitalis, used for dropsy (heart disease); and alcohol, used as a tranquilizer and as a treatment for a wide variety of illnesses for which no other therapy existed. Some drugs hastened death, some cured, and sometimes people recovered in spite of them. The strengths of the active substances in the drugs were undependable, as many were crude products from plant, animal, or mineral sources, not easily prepared.

Today drugs are monitored by the Food and Drug Administration (FDA). Early studies must be done on animals to determine a drug's toxicity, long-term effects, and side effects, and the results must be submitted to the FDA to warrant human studies. Several levels of studies on humans are then done to determine effectiveness, safety, dosage, and any long-term sequelae. Once a drug is approved by the FDA and is in clinical use, studies on its effects must continue (1, p. 5). The FDA also regulates labeling and can rule that clients must give informed consent for certain drugs. This is true of estrogen containing drugs, for example.

Since World War II, the pharmaceutical industry has virtually taken over the process of compounding medications, once the prerogative of pharmacists. This has resulted in the production of drugs that are consistent in dosage and quality (2, p.360). The impact of the pharmaceutical industry on health care is evident when one looks at the amount of money spent each year on prescription drugs: hospital and provider expenses head the list of costs, with drugs third. Although some of the insured do have coverage for prescription drugs, most do not. HMOs and other managed care groups often require a co-payment. Further, spending for prescription drugs does not take into account the millions of dollars people spend each year on over-the-counter preparations made by members of the Pharmaceutical Manufacturers Association (PMA) and hundreds of proprietary companies.

The pharmaceutical industry's contribution to drug research is significant. There are over 1,000 companies in the U.S. that handle or manufacture pharmaceuticals for human use. Of these, 93 belong to the PMA, which is responsible for 95% of prescription drugs sold here each year (3). These are called ethical drug companies because they don't advertise to the public. Members of the PMA spend millions of dollars a year on research (4), of which only a small portion goes for basic research. The rest of it is applied research, which is usually done with an eye toward increasing profits. Much applied research is done in medical schools, pharmacy schools, and hospitals. The National Institutes of Health also do a great deal of research.

When a new drug is developed, it is patented for 17 years, giving the company that produced it a monopoly on it for that period of time. Thus, although no member of the PMA controls a majority portion of the market, many have virtual monopolies on certain parts of that market (22). The patent in no way dictates price, so manufacturers can charge what they wish.

A new drug is given both a generic and a trade or brand name. The generic name, bestowed by a "naming group," is usually derived from the drug's chemical structure. The drug also has a chemical name which describes it exactly. The trade or brand name is coined by an advertising firm and is designed to trigger the memory and to catch attention. Thus, when writing a prescription, the physician or advanced practice nurse will be more likely to use the brand name. The provider's desk may boast a prescription pad on which the brand name of a drug (one the company may be especially promoting) is already imprinted. The provider need only indicate the quantity and sign the sheet. When the patent expires, other companies may produce the drug and they will give it their own brand name, or use the generic name. The original manufacturer has the edge because the product has become known by the original brand name.

Brand-name drugs are usually more costly than those with generic names. Thus it is that brand X of aspirin will cost more than acetylsalicylic acid. In recent years, many states have passed laws mandating that prescriptions be written in both generic and brand names. In addition, in many states pharmacies must now post prices of regularly used drugs comparing those for generic and brand-name products, must give prices over the telephone and/or must inform the consumer of any difference in prices. To stock both generic and brand-name drugs increases costs for the pharmacist, but it does offer choices to the consumer. It is legal, however, to fill a generic prescription with a brand-name drug, and that often occurs (5, p. 980).

High prices for brand-name drugs are justified by their manufacturers on the basis of costs for research and development, rink to the company if the drug causes problems for consumers, and costs of manufacturing and marketing. When a drug is under patent, competition is virtually nonexistent and the consumer has no choice but to pay. Drug companies argue that once patents have expired, there is free competition and prices drop.

It has also been argued that generic-name drugs are not as consistent in quality as brand-name products. FDA investigations have, thus far, failed to substantiate this claim (22).

The millions of prescriptions written for drugs each year attest to the power of the provider who writes those prescriptions. Prescription drugs account for 7-10% of the 835 billion dollars we spent for health care in 1992 (22). We have become a drug-oriented society. When someone describes a malady to us, we automatically respond with, "What are you taking for it?" or "What did your doctor/nurse practitioner prescribe?" We feel almost cheated if we visit a health care provider and are not given a prescription for something. The drug companies know this and use it to advantage. Pharmaceutical manufacturers employ detail persons whose job it is to entice providers to prescribe their products.

The industry as a whole spends several thousand dollars per year per physician for free samples, trade publications, advertising gimmicks, hospitality, detail persons' salaries (most are men), grants for research, courses, and gifts such as stethoscopes to medical students. Few similar gifts are bestowed upon nurses and nursing students or other providers, except those studying pharmacy who will have the power to dispense drugs. As nurses are empowered in more states to write or cosign prescriptions, we too are being courted by detail persons anxious to sell their products. Small wonder that the catchy brand name instantly flashes to a provider's consciousness when he or she writes a prescription—his or her office is decorated with reminders: pens, letter openers, anatomical models, journals, desk accoutrements, penlites, and drawers full of cleverly packaged samples. The wonders of the advertising world seem to blossom in all colors and shapes in the competition for the prescription writer's attention.

On an even more sobering note, the deluge of drugs and compounds, and the various types of drug dosages and strengths and forms (oral, injectable, topical, suppository)—thousands of drug entities and combinations and tens of thousands of dosage forms and strengths in all—is overwhelming. It should not be surprising, then, that providers rely too heavily at times on information from drug companies and their detail persons. Fortunately, pharmacists are becoming more vociferous and assertive, and generally keep drug records for all clients, and have increased their role as educators of clients and professionals. The neighborhood drug store, however, is being pushed out of business, however, by big drugstore chains, so the pharmacist may no longer know all his/her customers as once was the case.

Professional journals, the MEDLAR computer system of the National Library of Medicine, the American Medical Association's Department of Drugs, the FDA, and a number of reference books are available to aid prescribers. It should be noted that the well-known *Physician's Desk Reference* is distributed to physicians by the pharmaceutical industry and is paid for by members of the PMA. It should, therefore, be treated as one reference, but not as an authoritative source. *The United States Pharmacopoeia* and *The National Formulary* are the two official tomes for drug reference in this country. The FDA issues a monthly publication called the *FDA Drug Bulletin* which is available free of charge and is a source of information on hearings, warnings, and updates on old drugs and information on new ones.

Another of the disconcerting aspects of the pharmaceutical industry is the nature of its advertisements, particularly those relating to women. Peruse a medical journal of any sort and note the depictions of men and women in the drug ads. Also note how nurses are shown in the ads. Since physicians acknowledge that advertisements are important to them as sources of information on drugs, their content is not insignificant. In them, women are more often depicted as suffering from emotional illness and men from physical illness (6). Moreover, women are often shown in passive, dependent roles in relation to male physicians, as are nurses. The elderly, too, are often caricatured and demeaned (6).

In recent years, a new phrase has been added to our everyday vocabulary—"iatrogenic disease." Iatrogenic disease is that caused by therapy. Illnesses attributable to untoward reactions to drugs are only now beginning to be considered as important occurrences in the health system. One of the most glaring examples in recent times is the DES (diethylstilbestrol) scandal, which occurred after the discovery that a rare form of vaginal carcinoma in women occurred in those whose mothers had taken DES during pregnancy to prevent miscarriage. Another is the occurrence of serious and sometimes fatal anemias in people given chloramphenicol, an antibiotic. Yet another is the frequent occurrence of tardive dyskinesia in patients given phenothiazines, which are antipsychotic drugs. Still another example is the number of deaths and illnesses thought to be attributable to birth control pills.

All of these examples point out the risks and dangers directly attributable to drug therapy designed to treat a condition or, in the case of oral contraceptives, to prevent pregnancy. On the other hand, it is important to point out that such drugs as penicillin save countless lives, that drugs for tuberculosis virtually emptied the sanitoria, and that we need no longer fear a host of once fatal or debilitating diseases. Somehow a balance must be struck between the positive resources and research of the pharmaceutical industry and exploitation of the public.

Technology: Equipment and Supplies

The burgeoning of technological developments in this century has affected all aspects of our lives including health care. Americans spent nearly 48.9 billion dollars on drugs and health aids in 1990 (7). Unfortunately, most research and developmental work for medical equipment and devices takes place in commercial companies and not in the health community. Thus, devices may be unduly complex, expensive, or even unnecessary.

Disposables such as syringes, catheterization and enema sets, dietary utensils, dishes, emesis basins, urinals, bedpans, and even surgical drapes, gowns, masks, and gloves, are now available, and the list goes on and on. Whereas hospitals once had to concern themselves with the safe reprocessing of equipment, now they are confronted with the problem of what to do with all the waste generated by disposables. Moreover, much waste from health care agencies and institutions is biomedical hazardous waste and requires special handling. Because of AIDS, standards for employee protection have changed dramatically, as have regulations from CDC and other agencies to protect clients. Full compliance costs providers from thousands of dollars in private practice to millions for large hospitals.

At the same time, providers and consumers can rest considerably more comfortably with the assurance that needles and syringes are, indeed, sterile and that infant formulas are prepared properly. Morbidity and mortality from unsterile equipment, clogged syringes, sodium chloride in formulas, and unstable "in-house"-prepared intravenous solutions are, hopefully, part of history. However, quality control is now largely in the hands of manufacturers rather than in those of care providers, thus removing many of the technical aspects of care one step further away from the client. In some ways, this fact makes it all the more incumbent upon providrs to check la els carefully, note expiration dates and sterility indicators, and be generally cognizant of any irregularity in products. Grave and sometimes fatal errors have occurred becaues of similarities because of similarities in the appearance of products or because of their faulty assembly or preparation. In addition, the costs of equipment must be considered in planning and implementing care. Clients are often now billed for most equipment used in theii care. Disposable bed-protecting pads have replaced draw sheets and rubber sheets; clients are often charged for each pad used in their care. The advent of AIDS has created an immense market for protective products such as goggles, gloves, bins for used sharps, and for the safe handling and disposal of hazardous medical wastes, costs which are passed on to consumers.

Computing the cost effectiveness of using disposable versus reusable equipment is very complex. The initial cost of the reusable item plus its life expectancy must be computed along with the energy and personnel costs of washing, resterilizing, and preparing it for reuse. These costs must then be compared to the unit cost of the disposable item and personpower costs of unloading, storing, and delivering the item to the unit within the institution. Shelf life, storage space, and cost and method of disposal are also factors. Since many items are charged to the client, however, disposable items may well come out far ahead. Aside from the impact on the environment of tons of non-biodegradable wastes discarded by health care institutions each year, there is also the issue of what the use of these products does, in the long run, to health care costs. The practice of third party reimbursement only removes the burden from the client and transfers it to taxpayers or all those enrolled in the particular insurance plan. Ultimately we all pay. It is important to note that technological advances have made health care institutions safer places to be in when sick and have helped to transform them from places to go to die to places to go to recover. The point of this discourse is to encourage you as a provider and consumer within the system to be cognizant of the impact of disposable items on cost and on the environment and to be prepared to justify their use and contribution to quality health care. Moreover, AIDS has pushed us to use more disposables and to purchase and use expensive and sophisticated sterilizing equipment for nondisposable items.

Technology in health care, however, is scarcely limited to developing and manufacturing relatively simple disposable replacements for commonly used items. CAT (computerized axial tomography) or computed tomography (CT) scanners; magnetic resonance imaging (MRI); artificial hearts, hips, and knees; ultrasound; teleradiology; and all manner of monitors for body functions are but a few examples of developments within this century (8). All of these undoubtedly contribute much not only to the art and science of healing but also to the cost of health care. Technology also changes the way nursing care is delivered and places burdens on nurses who now have to care for patients *and* machines (24). The several thousand or million dollars each new piece of equipment costs an institution will ultimately be passed on to the consumer, either through direct use charges or through increased room rates, insurance premiums, or taxes.

One of the intentions of the Health Resources Planning and Development Act was to curb the acquisition of expensive equipment by each and every institution. This intention backfires when people complain that they have to travel 50 or 100 miles to have a particular treatment or test because their local community hospital cannot afford or has been denied permission to acquire the necessary equipment. Furthermore, hospitals and other health care institutions are anxious to have the latest and most sophisticated equipment in order to keep beds at full occupancy and to attract the best providers, especially physicians. Conflicts of interest arise, too, when physicians or other health care providers own diagnostic laboratories or stock in an equipment company.

Concern over the impact of medical technology on health care costs stimulated a forum, in 1977, devoted to that topic. Participants concluded that medical technology cannot be blamed for rising costs, and that the absence of incentives for cost control within the health care system are to blame for costs spiraling out of control. At the same time, however, they recommended that, to assure the safety and efficacy of technological advances, federal involvement must be expanded. That involvement should include gathering, assembling, evaluating, analyzing, and disseminating data related to technological advanced and procedures for health care (9).

The Office of Technology Assessment (OTA) is an arm of Congress designed to assist its members to understand changes in technology (8). With the formation of the Agency for Health Care Policy and Research, OTA was subsumed under its jurisdiction. A conference to examine innovative technologies was convened in 1992 (25).

Technology has also raised many moral and ethical dilemmas for health care providers. Sophisticated respirators and similar equipment have made possible the support of life when human resources fail. The deliberations of a Harvard ad hoc committee to spell out criteria for the presence of brain death represented one attempt to deal with critical ethical issues. The case of Karen Quinlan has become a classic in the fast-growing repertoire of medical excursions into the courts. In such cases, the question of quality of life becomes superimposed upon that of artificially sustaining life (10). Quality of life issues have become more critical in an age where we can keep people alive on life support systems for extended periods of time. The Advanced Directives Legislation at the federal and state levels (some states have living will or health care proxy legislation) exists to mandate and/or encourage us to consider our wishes when we are still able to do so (27).

Health Care as Big Business

There are, in the United States, more than 700 proprietary or for-profit hospitals with 100 or more beds and more than 20,000 rest, nursing, residential facilities, and convalescent homes, also run for profit (7). Whereas in 1939 there were 1,200 nursing homes in this country with 25,000 beds, less than 30 years later in 1967 (post-Medicare) there were I,I4I nursing homes with 846,544 beds (11). In the past nearly three decades the number of private, for-profit home health care and medical personnel agencies has increased drastically. Most cater to upper- and middle-income clients, shunning those who are poor. Exceptions to this are the nursing and convalescent homes, which are eager to harvest the fruits of Medicare and Medicaid and fill their beds to capacity with clients they know can pay through third-party payers. Resident facilities are also eager to court the approval of physicians upon whom they may be dependent for admissions, especially when a third party foots the bill and when utilization must be documented. Thus, physicians may be able to wield considerable power with these institutions. If they are dissatisfied with services, they can always send their clients elsewhere.

Nursing homes are of three types. The majority of them offer nursing care; a small number offer personal care with some nursing; and about a quarter offer only personal care. In order for most third-party payers to cover the cost, the client must require nursing care. The vast majority of clients are women over 80 years of age. Seventy-five percent of nursing homes are proprietary, 5% are government supported, and only 20% are nonprofit (7). The advent of Medicare and Medicaid was a boon to nursing homes. The original Social Security Act provided old age assistance funds and retirement benefits for older Americans, but not for those in institutions (12, pp. I24-I25). Prior to the forties, the poor were cared for in almshouses, county poor farms and, in some cases, church supported homes. In I950, amendments to the Social Security Act provided monies for care in public facilities (I3). Since then, restrictions require the client (or spouse) to be all but impoverished in order for Medicare/Medicaid to pay.

Care in nursing homes ranges from good to marginal to down-right poor. Of the 30 million Americans over 65, only 1% of those from age 65-74 are in long-term care institutions but 22% of those 85 and older are. In a comparative study of persons over 65 in long-term institutions in Scotland and in the U.S., the quality of care was found to be significantly better in Scotland. Furthermore, residents of such institutions in Scotland were allowed more choices and more freedom and independence than residents in similar institutions in the U.S. (14).

As of 1966, the Joint Commission on Accreditation of Health Care Organizations (JCAHO) has assumed responsibility for accrediting nursing homes and convalescent, extended, and resident care facilities (12, p. 125). Criteria for long-term care facilities have been developed under the JCAHO (26). Such facilities must meet Medicaid and Medicare standards to be certified for reimbursement by those plans. States also license nursing homes. Medicare coverage is limited in amount and in the number of days covered, with the client paying some of the costs. The client may also be eligible for Medicaid funds, or he or she may have some other insurance which will cover all or part of the costs not assumed under Medicare. However, costs are high and many cannot afford those homes which offer high quality care. About 50% of the cost of long-term care is paid by patients.

Serious abuse of clients in some nursing homes has come to light in recent years. Triggered by the incentive to make money, some operators cut costs to a minimum or refuse Medicaid clients because Medicaid pays a per diem rate (15).

Some authors claim that the majority of nursing homes are substandard or at least border on neglect. They assert that most are unsafe (16; 17, pp. 155-156). Others point out the positive aspects of the intimate social ties that may develop and the positive sharing that may occur between the residents and staff of a nursing home (18, 29).

Although not all nursing homes are either neglectful or abusive, even one case is significant because it represents disrespect for human life. Given the number of nursing homes in the country, it is an almost impossible task for cities, states, the federal government, and accrediting bodies to monitor the care closely enough to detect all the neglect and abuse that may occur. It is incumbent upon individual providers to expose instances of clients being deprived of care, nutrition, or the services to which they are entitled and for which they or the third party are paying.

A phenomenon in health care is its development as a major new industry. Corporate-owned hospitals, nursing homes, clinics, HMOs, home care agencies, free-standing medical, surgical, and dialysis centers, managed care organizations, and even medical practices are becoming common. One corporation owns hundreds of hospitals. There are over 500 listed corporations competing for health care investment dollars. Of these, the largest diversified companies own over 11% of community hospitals and 66% of nursing homes and chronic care facilities. Corporations are also major purchasers of health care, largely through employee benefit packages, and now spend over 125 billion dollars a year; 54% of private employees are now covered by managed care plans compared to 5% in 1980 (20, 27). Thus, to say health care is big business is an understatement. In 1993, however, with shorter lengths of stay and incentives in managed care to keep people out of hospitals, occupancy rates are down and hospitals are closing units and laying off personnel, many of them nurses (21).

Home Care Agencies

Until very recently, the preponderance of home care was provided through official health agencies (public health departments), visiting nursing associations, and hospital programs. Most of these services are approved for Medicare reimbursement (12, p. 126). With the monies Medicare has made available for home care, however, proprietary agencies have begun to vie for their piece of the pie. Such agencies may provide both skilled nursing and/or homemaker services for visits ranging from once a week to several hours each day. They may employ registered nurses, licensed practical nurses, and/or home health or homemaker aides. The latter may be former nurses' aides or may receive a training course ranging from days to weeks. Some agencies also employ nursing students.

Home care can be less costly than hospital or nursing home care (17). As important to consider as the cost, however, are the benefits to patients and the family and friends caring for them. It is difficult to coordinate home care so as to assure continuity among a variety of providers. It is also difficult to assure quality care, particularly when care is provided by an agency interested in profit and not monitored in any way except for Medicare regulations and state licensure. Persons needing home care may live alone and thus there is no family member there to monitor the care given. When proprietary agencies work in close collaboration with public health departments or visiting nurse services, some assessment of quality of care is easier to obtain. What is most frightening is the lack of preparation of home health or homemaker aides, who are often literally hired off the street, and the lack of commitment to clients who depend upon the services of these aides. As persons are discharged earlier and sicker from hospitals, home care has shifted from rehabilitation to illness care and even critical care. One proprietary home care agency in the Northeast categorized as a critical care agency employs 2,200 persons and grossed 233 million dollars in 1991 (23).

On the other hand, homemaker services can augment clients' own abilities and allow them to remain at home. A result of DRGs and short hospital stays is large numbers of ill persons at home with monitors, intravenous equipment, and even respirators who desperately need homemaker services. Unfortunately, eligibility restrictions for third-party payment have tightened dramatically, so that home care is very limited in amount and duration. As providers and consumers, we can support legislation to monitor and regulate proprietary home health care agencies so the level of care is appropriate and the client is a beneficiary rather than a victim.

Personnel Services

As our health care system continues to be plagued by a maldistribution of providers, numerous proprietary staffing agencies have emerged. Once concerned primarily with providing private duty nurses, and operating on a nonprofit basis, these "Kelly Girl" agencies for nursing are now big business. They find employment for nurses and other health care workers. For a fee they arrange with hospitals and other agencies to provide the workers required. Several of these advertise regularly in our journals. TravCorps®, Cross Country Healthcare®, Medical Express®, Resource Mobile Corps®, Circulating Nurses Division®, Med Staff®, and American Mobile Nurses® are a few of these agencies.

These service agencies may be independently owned or part of national corporations with many branches. So far, they are not licensed or regulated by any level of government or by professional groups. Disconcertingly, personnel may be used not only for supplementary, private duty and vacation or weekend coverage, but also as *total* staffing for units (21). This has been exacerbated by continuing nursing shortages in some areas.

The reasons given for choosing to work for an agency seem to center on control. Young nurses, eager to earn money and relatively unconcerned about benefits for retirement, may opt for agency employment. So employed, they can name their hours, units, days off, shifts, and agency, and can avoid weekend duty and some of the staffing hassles of hospitals while earning the same take-home pay as other nurses, albeit perhaps minus benefits. If they work for one of the travel nurse agencies, they can travel.

There is concern among nurses employed directly by health care agencies that the quality of care provided by personnel agency nurses is lower than that of the nurses employed by health care agencies. Means of evaluation and control also seem to be lacking. In addition, these personnel agencies affect hospital morale and the ability of hospitals to recruit and retain staff. Some moves are being made now by professional organizations to develop policy statements, regulations, and standards for such agencies. There are also attempts to formalize relationships between personnel agencies and health care institutions. In addition, there is a need to integrate nurses employed by these agencies into the system so they are subject to both its rewards and sanctions. Some important questions must be answered and issues addressed so that the integrity and reputation of professional nursing are retained and fostered and the client does not, once more, become the victim.

Summary

In understanding the complexity of our health care system, it is important to recognize the role private enterprise plays. Without denying the importance of the capitalistic spirit to democracy, one must also exercise caution. Every facet of life has its profiteers and the health care system is no exception. As providers and consumers of that system, we can act both as client advocates and as informed voters. The lobbying power we each possess can influence public policy on matters concerned with the proprietary enterprises in health care so that consumers are protected, and so that we are not obligated to support those industries which are exploitive. Finally, we can assist in exposing cases of overt abuse, neglect, and exploitation of clients. Lest you think that is beyond your ability to accomplish, let us assure you it is not. Only a few years ago, two of our students collected data on safety hazards in nursing homes in their local area. Once they had collected sufficient data, they presented it to persons of authority concerned with nursing home licensure and eventually testified before the Senate Committee on Aging. They have also published their results. So each of us can influence what goes on within the system, if only in a small way.

References

1. Asperheim, M.K. and Eisenhauer, L.A. (1977). The Pharmacologic Basis of Patient Care, 3rd ed. Philadelphia: W.B. Saunders.
2. Mrtek, R.G. (1976). Pharmaceutical education in these United States: An interpretive historical essay of the twentieth century. American Journal of Pharmaceutical Education 40:339-365.
3. Dun's Million $ Disc. (1993): Dun's Marketing Services, Inc.
4. Basic Data Relating to the National Institutes of Health. (1976). Washington, DC: National Institutes of Health.
5. Gumbhir, A.K. and Rodowskas, C.A. (1974). Consumer price differentials between generic and brand name prescriptions. American Journal of Public Health 64(10):977-982.
6. Hawkins, J.J., and Aber, C.S. (1993). Women in advertisements in medical journals. Sex Roles 28(3-4):228-242.
7. Statistical Abstract of the United States 1992, 112th ed. (1992). Washington, CD: U.S. Department of Commerce, Bureau of the Census.
8. McCormick, K.A. (1983). Preparing nurses for the technological future. Nursing and Health Care 4(7):379-382.
9. Altman, S.H. and Blendon, R., eds. (1979). Medical Technology: The

Culprit Behind Health Care Costs? Proceedings of the 1977 Sun Valley Forum on National Health, p.302. Washington, DC: U.S. Government Printing Office.

10. Reiser, S.J. (1977). Therapeutic choice and moral doubt in a technological age. In: J.H. Knowles, ed., Doing Better and Feeling Worse. New York: W.W. Norton, pp. 47-56.
11. Freymann, J.G. (1974). The American Health Care System: Its Genesis and Trajectory. New York: MEDCOM Press, p. 31.
12. Wilner, D.M., Walkley, R.B., and O'Neill, E.J. (1978). Introduction to Public Health, 7th ed. New York: Macmillan.
13. Thomas, W.C. (1969). Nursing Homes and Public Policy. Ithaca, NY: Cornell University Press, p. 7.
14. Kayser-Jones, J. (1979). Care of the institutionalized aged in Scotland and the United Sates: A comparative study. Western Journal of Nursing Research 1(3):190-193.
15. Hochbaum, M. and Galkin, F. (1987). Medicaid patients need not apply. Social Policy 17(4):40-42.
16. Mendelson, M. (1974). Tender Loving Greed. New York: Knopf.
17. Kemper, P., Applebaum, R. and Harrigan, M. (1987). Community care demonstrations: What have we learned? Health Care Financing Review 8(4):87-100.
18. Gubrium, J.F. (1975). Living and Dying at Murray Manor. New York: St. Martin's Press.
19. Subcommittee on Long Term Care, Special Committee on Aging, U.S. Senate. (1974). Nursing Home Care in the U.S.: Failure of Public Policy. Supporting Paper No. 1. Washington, DC: U.S. Government Public Office.
20. Miller, I. (1984). The Health Care Survival Curve: Competition and Cooperation in the Marketplace. Homewood, IL: Dow Jones-Irwin.
21. Noble, B.P. (1993, Jan. I0). Pushing nurses to a breaking point. The New York Times, p. 25.
22. Pharmaceutical companies under fire. (1993). A.S.A.P. 9(1):3.
23. Bloomsberg Business News, 1993.
24. Pillar, B., Jacox, A.K. and Redman, B.K. (1990). Technology, its assessment, and nursing. Nursing Outlook 38(1):16-19.
25. Grady, M.L. (1992). New Medical Technology: Experimental or State-of-the-art. Rockville, MD: Agency for Health Care Policy and Research.
26. Joint Commission on Accreditation for Hospital Organizations. (1992). Accreditation Manual for Long Term Care. Chicago: JCAHO.
27. Patient self-determination act regulations remain at HCFA. (1991). Capital Update 9(22):7.
28. Why wait for Hillary? (June 28, 1993). Newsweek, 38-40.
29. Retsinas, J. (1986). It's OK, Mom. The Nursing Home from a Sociological Perspective. New York: The Tiresias Press.

9

Models for Health Care Delivery: Experiences in Other Countries

The United States is the only industrialized country in the world besides South Africa that does not have a national health service or a plan of national health insurance. It is the intention of this chapter to explore several models from other countries as examples of alternatives to the private-enterprise-dominated system we have in the United States. It is not our intention to advocate any of the systems presented, but rather to describe and examine them for components that might be useful as we contemplate a restructuring of our present modes of health care delivery.

World Systems

There are three predominant systems of health care delivery. The first of these, dominate in roughly 108 countries, is that of *public assistance*. The countries with this system are in Asia, Africa, and Latin America, and might be termed second- or third-world developing nations. In the second system, a *national health insurance* scheme is in place. Approximately 23 countries, including those in Western

Europe and North America, as well as Australia, New Zealand, Japan, and Israel have such plans. For example, Germans must enroll in one of 1,100 sickness funds, similar to our nonprofit Blue Cross-Blue Shield; coverage is funded by a payroll tax shared by employers and employees (27). In the United States, private insurance predominates, whereas in Canada, Denmark, Finland, Iceland, New Zealand, and Norway everyone is covered by a national government health insurance plan, although in New Zealand there is some movement toward a competitive market system. The third system in found in the 14 countries with *national health services*: nine are socialist countries in Europe, four are in Asia, and the other one is Cuba. Of course, with the dramatic changes in Eastern Europe, an unraveling of some of the systems is occurring. The decade of the 1990s will witness changes there as well as in other parts of the world. Terris identifies Sweden and the United Kingdom as countries that have components of both national health insurance and national health service (1).

The countries chosen for discussion in this chapter represent some variations in evolution and implementation of the plans as well as differences in population and geographic characteristics. Their similarities to and differences from the U.S. system make their inclusion significant in an analysis of our present system, offering as they do some possibilities for change in our system. (See Table 9.1.)

The United Kingdom

England's Poor Law Act of 1601 mandated that local authorities provide for the sick, needy, and homeless. In 1848, the Public Health Act established a comprehensive public health system. The National Health Insurance Act of 1912 established a plan whereby all persons earning less than 150£ a year (later, 420£) could have the services of a general practitioner. Financing was done through employee and employer contributions to insurance societies. This plan covered about half of the population: the rest of the people were responsible for their own care through fee for service or private insurance societies. In 1944, a comprehensive national health service was proposed and two years later the National Health Service Act was

Table 9.1   A Comparison of the Structure of Health Systems in Five Selected Countries.

Country	Type	Method of Payment	Copayment	Services Provided	Administered by
United States	private insurance; some government involvement	fee for service; private insurance premiums; federal coverage for selected groups; general taxes, s.s taxes	many	hospitalization; some e.r.; ambulatory; nursing home	private companies; social security admin.; welfare organ.; state and federal
United Kingdom	national health service	health and social security payments deducted from pay; general taxation	some	primary care hospital; specialist care; home care; nursing home care	Dept. of Health and Social Security
Canada	national health insurance	sharing federal/ provincial; income tax surcharge; general revenues; premiums; % of payroll	some	medical, hospital care; cash sickness and maternity benefits; nursing home care (some)	Dept. of National Health and Welfare; provincial governments
Sweden	national health insurance; components of national health service	municipal and county councils, the State; the insured; contributions from employers' payroll taxes	some	medical, hospital care; cash benefits for illness, maternity; nursing home; ambulance; home care; dental care	Ministry of Health and Social Affairs, National Board of Health and Welfare
China	national health service	central government through Chinese Communist Party	none	all services	Ministry of Health

passed, to commence operation in 1948 (2, pp. 1-2).

In 1982, the National Health Service was reorganized. The two-tier structure divided the country into 14 Regional Health Authorities, each containing at least one university medical school. The Regional Health Authorities were responsible for regional health planning, provision of services, allocation of resources to district health authorities (DHAs), quality assurance of the DHAs, and support of teaching and research in universities.

The DHAs assess health needs in their districts and plan, organize, and administer district health services. The DHAs consist of appointed but unpaid lay and professional citizens. Their executive arm is the District Management Team. Each health district has a population of about 250,000 people (15, 16).

Covered under the National Health Service are public health responsibilities for water supply, sewage disposal, clean air, good housing, control of infectious diseases and food poisoning, immigration and quarantine, immunization, pure food, safe medicines, and laboratory services, as well as such miscellaneous local concerns as refuse disposal, street cleaning, and burial grounds (2, pp. 8-12).

Health services to individuals include: primary care (50% of physicians are general practitioners); hospital and specialist care; special programs for mothers, children, the elderly, the chronic sick, the disabled, and the mentally ill; and concern for occupational safety and health (2, pp. 16-35). There is much emphasis on home care, especially for elders (29).

Costs of the National Health Service are borne in part by Health and Social Security payments deducted from the pay of all workers, but the greater portion of funds comes from general taxation (3). Whereas at first all services were free, many services now require partial payment by the client. For example, clients must pay part of the costs of dental care, glasses, prescriptions, and so on. Some persons are eligible under law for free services, but many must pay at least some of the costs of care (2, pp. 14-20). People may also opt for private care (16, 29), and about 10% have private insurance.

Conditions affecting the salaries and employment of National Health Service workers are settled between providers and government administrators at the national level. Thus, nurses' salaries are the same in all parts of the country. Differentials are recognized for certain services such as "on call," overtime, and certain specialties (3). Each DHS has its own school of nursing; the General Nursing Councils oversee curricula. Nursing education includes four basic three-year programs: general, pediatric, psychiatric, and mental handicap. Programs within universities or polytechnics are growing in number as nursing education begins a slow move to universities and to a research base for practice.

Problems have arisen in the British scheme. Those at the bottom rung of the socioeconomic ladder—the homeless—do not always have health care, although financial barriers are absent. Concerted efforts to reach homeless persons have been successful, however, demonstrating that creative problem solving can work (28). Resources are insufficient to meet demands for services: facilities are rundown, equipment is in short supply, there is a shortage of nurses, and the waiting time, especially for elective services, can be very long. Malpractice, too, has begun to show up for British physicians, who once considered themselves immune. Private health care, although increasing, accounts for only a small percent of spending. An estimated five and a half million persons have private health insurance, and there are about 200 private hospitals and a few for profit (30). The National Health Service is one of Europe's biggest employers, having one million persons on its payroll (23, 24, 25).

The British system, although far from ideal, nonetheless offers one model for making health services available to all, attempting to regulate costs, access, and the distribution of services and providers, and planning and providing health care at the national level. The British spend only 6% of their GNP on health care (29), slightly less than $1,300 per capita. The system has dealt, albeit not perfectly, with rationing of care, an issue facing the U.S. today (10, 23). Interestingly, while we examine alternative models for health care delivery in the U.S., proposals are being made in Great Britain to encourage competition, adopt elements of privatization, and make changes in the way general practitioners and specialists practice (30).

Canada

The Canadian system can trace its origins to the province of Saskatchewan where, in 1914, one of the rural municipalities formed a medical care insurance program funded by taxes. The province then passed a law permitting municipal governments to do this, and in 1917 another law was passed permitting support for hospital care as well. Other provinces did likewise. It was not until 1961, however, that all provinces had national health insurance for hospital costs, and not until the early 1970s that all provinces and territories came under the aegis of the Medical Care Act of 1966 (5, pp. 23-25), amended by Bill C-3 passed by the House of Commons, April 9, 1984 (22).

The Department of National Health and Welfare is the major agency at top government level responsible for health. The Health Programs Branch is responsible for administering the federal share of the provinces' hospital and medical insurance costs, for acting in a technical advisory capacity, and for providing health personpower training assistance and health research grants. The involvement at the federal level in actual health care delivery is very limited since health care delivery is the responsibility of the ten provinces and regional and local authorities. The mode of organization for health care delivery varies among the provinces (5, p. 25).

Coverage includes medical, dental, and hospital care, and most workers are eligible for cash sickness and maternity benefits as well. Glasses, ambulance fees, hearing aids, medical appliances, and prescription drugs are not covered, although some of the provinces include care by other providers. Many residents carry private nonprofit insurance for benefits not covered (5, pp. 27-29; 22). The 1984 act includes a clause on extended health care services: nursing home care, adult residential care, home care, and ambulatory care.

The cost of coverage under the Federal Medical Care Act is shared by the federal government and the provinces. The federal government's share is financed through a percentage income tax surcharge. The provinces' share comes from general revenues, and some of the provinces charge a premium. Employers also contribute a percentage of payroll in some provinces. Low income residents are exempt from paying premiums (5, pp. 32-32). Health care costs are lower per capita in Canada than in the United States and use a smaller percentage of the gross national product, at less than 9% (6, 32). Administrative costs in the United States are $95 per capita versus $21 (Canadian) in Canada, according to a General Accounting Office study (31).

In three provinces, worker-controlled occupational health centers have been established. These appear to provide a useful model for focusing on work-place hazards and for altering occupational health practice patterns (26, pp. 692-693).

Nursing services are critical to delivery of health care in a country as large as Canada with a sparse and scattered population. Nursing began its outreach in organized health care with missionary services, and later within the organization of the government health services. Access to health care for residents in remote areas is, in large part, dependent upon nurses. Hundreds of field nurses serve north of the 60th parallel (8, pp. 481-487; 31). Nurse practitioners have found little acceptance in Canada other than in the far north and Newfoundland where their tradition is legendary. This is probably due to adequate supplies of physicians in most provinces (9, p. 888; 31) and, possibly, to a perceived challenge to medical dominance. By 1992, 150-200 nurses across Canada belonged to the Nurse Practitioner Association of Ontario (31).

Providers are reimbursed by the provinces. Private duty nursing services, if not covered by the national scheme, are covered and reimbursed by private companies; nurses as primary care providers are reimbursed by some provincial and territorial health insurance plans through the health services. Nurses are employed by hospitals, the majority of which are public, municipal, or provincial, or by agencies in more populated areas, and are salaried. Salary limits occur through cost control mechanisms designed to curb escalating health care costs (9, pp. 885-888).

Problems within the Canadian system include escalating costs, physician discontent with set fees resulting in a trend toward extra billing for charges beyond what is reimbursed, disregard for costs by providers, government control of the supply and distribution of medical specialists, and reluctance to introduce other health care providers such as advanced practice nurses to the system (9, pp. 887-889; 7, pp. 30-31; 37). However, the system has weathered economic and energy crises well, it is intact, its costs are far less than those in the United States, and by conventional measures, Canadians are healthier than white Americans (9, pp. 888-889). Although we would scarcely suggest that the Canadian scheme be transplanted intact to this country, it does offer one example of a system that works in a country with a government similar to ours, a physician fee for service practice, and reliance on third-party reimbursement.

Sweden

Voluntary health insurance funds have existed in Sweden since 1850. Government involvement began with registering such funds in 1891 and with public supervision in 1910. By 1935, the voluntary program was open to all in good health from ages 15 to 50, and there were no age restrictions in group plans. The program was financed by premiums paid by workers, with the government contributing 20%. Then in 1955 the compulsory universal health insurance plan was introduced to cover all citizens (5, p. 80).

The national insurance system administers not only health coverage, but old age and disability benefits as well through 26 regional offices corresponding with county geographic regions. Each of these has a catchment area of 60,000 to 1,500,000 people, with an average of 300,000 (33). These offices are supervised by the National Social Insurance Board. The major federal agency for health is the National Board of Health and Welfare, a component of the cabinet-level ministry of Health and Social Affairs. Control of all medical care resides with the national government, but responsibility for care delivery is in the hands of county councils. Organization is four-level: a regional hospital for an area population of one to 1.5 million, where the superspecialties are concentrated in six medical care regions; county hospitals of 800 to 1,000 beds serving 250,000 to 300,000 people; local district hospitals with fewer than 300 beds serving 60,000 to 90,000 people; and some 300 local health centers throughout the country which provide 5,000 to 50,000 people with ambulatory care (11, 36).

Coverage for both medical and hospital care is available for all residents. Cash benefits are also paid for illness and maternity time for those who are employed. There is some cost sharing for certain medications and dental care. Nursing homes, day care, and home health care are provided, as is ambulance service (5, pp. 84-86; 35). Financing is accomplished through the municipal and county councils, employers, and the insured (34).

Most hospitals and other inpatient and ambulatory facilities are owned and operated by the county councils, which are thus the chief employers of physicians and other health care workers. Most of the physicians in Sweden are specialists, and the majority of these are public employees. District medical offices in rural and outlying areas are often staffed by public health nurses and midwives, who provide primary care. Because most facilities are operated by the counties, most nurses are also public employees. These providers are salaried on fee schedules. Pharmacies are also controlled and operated by a state monopoly (5, pp. 81-83,89; 36).

Problems inherent in the Swedish system include economics and the impersonal nature of the system, including waits for care and, in some cases, lack of humane and adequate care for elders (37). Escalating costs have made it necessary to close and consolidate hospital facilities, especially those under 400 beds, and to create super-hospitals where specialists are concentrated. The social bureaucracy and highly structured system remove some of the personal aspects of care (11, pp. 132-135). Nonetheless, this system presents some important lessons that could profitably be learned by the United States. Some of the cost control mechanisms that are successfully applied in Sweden might be used here. Although geographically dissimilar, the two nations do share prosperity and a high degree of industrialization. Prototypes of mergers of small hospitals, consolidation of services such as maternity, and shared support services (laundries, clinical laboratories) are worthy of study for application here (11, pp. 136-141). It is not necessary that we adopt a complete system in order to benefit from its expertise in selected areas (24).

China

Prior to 1949, China was plagued by epidemics of communicable diseases, famine, and drug addiction. It had few medical facilities and providers, and poor or nonexistent public health measures. Before the Cultural Revolution in the late 1960s, quality medical care was scarce, medical centers few, and only those who could afford care had access to it. After the Cultural Revolution of the late 1960s, however, a tiered system reaches virtually every household (12, p. 40).

The rural medical system begins with a health station ("production brigade health station") staffed by a "paramedic" with six months to two years of training (many are women), health aides, and midwives (27, 38). The paramedics are the famous "barefoot doctors," a term dropped in 1984 and replaced by the term "rural doctors" (who passed an exam). A communal hospital forms the next level. This is a health facility or hospital of modest size with some beds for inpatients. It is staffed by Western and traditional doctors, nurses, and other health care providers. A more sophisticated facility ("central commune hospital"), run by a municipality, county, prefecture, or province, forms the next tier. At this level, there are also specialty hospitals for tuberculosis, mental illness, leprosy, and so on. There is a subdivision of the health care delivery system for each political subdivision in the administration of China. Thus there are communal hospitals and health care facilities; central commune hospitals with more sophisticated facilities; and provincial, municipal, and county hospitals. Although this sounds very structured, county systems vary and there are diverse functions and facilities in the tiers. Some rely on traditional medicine and others are almost exclusively Westernized (38).

Communes are divided into production brigades of a few thousand persons, served by health stations. These brigades are divided into production teams of several hundred persons who are served by a variety of professional and nonprofessional health care providers. Those at the bottom level of the production team may have responsibility for certain aspects of health care, public health, or sanitation, while also working in agriculture or industry (12, pp. 39-40). Interspersed in the system are folk practitioners, herbalists, and Western modes of care. China is an example of a country where indigenous medicine and cosmopolitan medicine are well-integrated. There are over 500,000 personnel involved in traditional medical services (38).

Because of the nature of the governmental structure, the private enterprise system is nonexistent; all health care workers are employees of the state and benefits are extended to all Chinese, but insurance coverage varies by occupation (18).

The costs of health care are borne primarily by the production teams, brigades, communes, factories, or counties (17). Priorities are set by the Ministry of Health. At present, these priorities include family planning, immunization, control of infectious diseases, occupational health, improved sanitation, and maternal and child nutrition and care (13, 19). Family planning has such a high priority that most Chinese women use the pill or intrauterine devices, and abortions and sterilizations are performed by aides, "rural doctors," and other paramedics (14, p. 665).

Health care providers are trained by the government and work for the government. A person's career as a health care professional depends upon the needs of the people, the recommendations of the community, and administrative screening. There seems to be little free choice. There are about 450 formal nursing schools with two- or three-year programs, supplemented by continuing or specialty education. Schools are at the trade-school level. Graduation from middle school is required. Since 1982, China has been moving toward university-based nursing education (17, 21).

The limitations of the system include a lack of freedom for providers, the cost and difficulty of travel, priority setting by the communist committee, a stigma attached to mental illness, and a lack of uniformity in training paramedical workers (13, 18, 12, p. 44). It is, however, impressive to consider a system that reaches virtually all the inhabitants of a country so vast but so rural and agricultural in much of its development, and which emphasizes prevention and serving the workers and demonstrates excellence in selected areas. It has much to teach those countries where costly drugs and technology are heavily relied upon.

In the late 1980s, China shifted to a system which allowed workers to share in profits over a certain level of production. Accompanying this economic shift was a decrease in the effectiveness of the one family/one child rule together with increased worker productivity and a demand for improved health services with a focus on curative needs (27).

Summary

The United Kingdom, Canada, Sweden, and China each represent different modes of organizing, delivering, and paying for health care. The differences between these nations in geography, population, culture, government, and social organization are striking. Each health care delivery system has, however, one or more components similar to one or more components of our system, and each system has facets that are worthy of evaluation in relation to our own. As the wealthiest nation, we have the potential for the best health care system. To accomplish this will require more than the present Band Aid approach. In restructuring the system, we can profit from the experience of countries that are pioneers in adapting national schemes and making them work.

References

1. Terris, M. The Three World Systems of Medical Care: Trends and Prospects. (1978.) *American Journal of Public Health*:68:11:1125-1131.
2. *Health Services in Britain.* 1974. London: Her Majesty's Stationery Office.
3. Nuttall, P.D. The British National Health Service.(1977.) *Nursing Outlook*:25:2:98-102.
4. Brown, R. G. S. *The Changing National Health Service.* 1973. London: Routledge and Kegan Paul.
5. *National Health Systems in Eight Countries.* 1975. Washington, DC: U. S. Department of Health, Education, and Welfare, Social Security Administration, Office of Research and Statistics.

6.   Greenberg, S. All Canadians Assured of Medical Care. (January 4,1976.) *Providence Sunday Journal:* C-1:6

7.   Glaser, W. A. *Health Insurance Bargaining.* 1978. New York: Gardner Press.

8.   Keith, C. W.Leadership in Nursing North of Sixty. (1971.)*Nursing Clinics of North America:*6:3:479-488.

9.   Hatcher, G. H. Canadian Approaches to Health Policy Decisions: National Health Insurance. (1978.) *American Journal of Public Health:*68:9:881-889.

10. The NHS: 40 Years Serving the Public. (1988). *The Health Service Journal Supplement,* 30 June: 3-22.

11. Government Policy and Women's Health Care: The Swedish Alternative. (1988). *Women & Health:* 13 (3/4), entire issue.

12. Axelrod, L. and A. Leaf. Aesculapius in China. (1976.) *Harvard Magazine:*79:3:38-44.

13. Mechanic, D. and A. Kleinman. Ambulatory Medical Care in the People's Republic of China: An Exploratory Study. (1980.) *American Journal of Public Health:*70:1:62:66.

14. Taeuber, I. B. Public Health and Demographic Transition in the People's Republic of China. (1977.) *American Journal of Public Health:*67:7:664-667.

15. Nuttall, P.D. British Nursing—Beginning of a Power Struggle. (1983). *Nursing Outlook:* 31:3:184-187.

16. Chaplin, N. *Getting It Right? The 1982 Reorganization of the National Health·Service.* 1982. London: Institute of Health Service Administrators.

17. Liu, Y.C. *China: Health Care in Transition.* (1983). *Nursing Outlook:* 31:2:94-99.

18. Henderson, G.E., and M.S. Cohen. Health Care in the People's Republic of China: A View from inside the System. (1982). *American Journal of Public Health:* 72:11:1238-1245.

19. Christiani. D.C. Occupational Health in the People's Republic of China. (1982). *American Journal of Public Health:* 74:1:58-64.

20. Hinman, A.R., R.L. Parker, G. Xue-gi, G. Xing-yuan, Y. Xi-fu, and H. De-yu. Health Services in Shanghai County. (1982). *American Journal of Public Health:* 72:95.

21. Drischel, K.M. Teaching Nursing in China—an Exchange Program. (1981). *Nursing Outlook:* 29:12:722-725.

22. The House of Commons of Canada. *Bill C-3.* (1984). Ottawa, Canada: Canadian Government Publishing Center.

23. British Health Service is Ailing and Thatcher has a Remedy in Mind. (1988). *The Wall Street Journal:* 211:37:1, 13.

24. Malpractice Virus is Showing Up in Britain. (1988). *The Boston Globe:* 233:33-34.

25. British Health System Faces Midlife Crisis. (1988). *The Boston Globe:* 233:18:1,3.

26. Yassi, A. The Development of Worker-Controlled Occupational Health Center in Canada. (1988). *American Journal of Public Health:* 78:6:689-693.

27. Germany's health-care model. (1991, May 5). *The Boston Sunday Globe*, p. 88.

28. Reuler, J.B. (1989). Health care for the homeless in a national health program. *American Journal of Public Health* 79:1033-1035.

29. Whittington, R.M. (1993). Crises in health care: United States and United Kingdom. *VA Practitioner* 10(2):47-48, 53.

30. Vall-Spinosa, A. (1991). Lessons from London: The British are reforming their national health service. *American Journal of Public Health* 81(12):1566-1570.

31. Van der Horst, M. (1992). Canada's health care system provides lessons for NPs. *The Nurse Practitioner* 17(8):44,50,52-53,57,60.

32. Marmor, J.R. and Mashaw, J.L. (1991). Canada's health insurance and ours: Real lessons, big choices. *The National Voter* 40(5):10-11.

33. *Swedish Legislation on Health and Medical Care.* (1990). Stockholm, Sweden: Ministry of Health and Social Affairs.

34. The cost of financing of the social services in Sweden in 1990. (1992). *Statistics Sweden.*

35. The care of the elderly in Sweden. (1992). *Fact Sheets on Sweden.*

36. Health and Medical care in Sweden. (1991). *Fact Sheets on Sweden.*

37. Bergström, H. (1992). Pressures behind the Swedish health reforms. *Viewpoint Sweden* #12.

38. Phillips, D.R. (1990). *Health and Health Care in the Third World.* New York: Longman Scientific & Technical.

10

Solutions and Alternatives

A health care system does not exist in a vacuum.* After decades of discussions about the pros and cons of a national health care system, many forces have converged that virtually guarantee fundamental changes in the way that health care is delivered and financed in the United States. Among the reasons for the national consensus on the need for health care reform are runaway costs, large numbers of Americans not covered by health insurance, health insurance tied to employment, and the uninsurability of people with certain diseases or preexisiting conditions.

A health care system requires the nurture of a climate influenced by political ideologies, economics, scientific discoveries, technological advances, and broad world events. Therefore, as an alternative to forecasting, we would like to propose a goal. This goal, unreachable perhaps, is a perfect health care system. Two limitations are inherent in such a goal. First, not everyone would agree on what a "perfect" health care system would consist of. Second, because of the changing nature of our society, that which looks good today may seem flawed tomorrow. With these limitations in mind, we will describe a utopian system embodying philosophy and action as a goal. We shall then discuss some current trends in ethics, organization, science and technology, and nursing.

---

* The interacting variables that have shaped the present system will also affect the solutions to its problems.

Health Care Utopia — 2000 A.D.

The ideal health care system will combine the best of scientific discovery and the highest level of philosophical thought. Those who need care will receive it. Because citizens will be knowledgeable about their bodies and feel in control of them, and because they will be assured of care when need occurs, there will be no abuse of the system. Health education as a form of primary preventive intervention will be considered a major subject and will be begun when a child enters school. Because people will understand and respect their bodies, the abuse of such substances as tobacco, alcohol, and drugs will have decreased dramatically. Mental health will be considered important and school programs will be geared toward strengthening students' self-esteem. That the total program works will be apparent in the decline of the incidence of adolescent pregnancies, school absences, and vandalism.

One of the most important areas that will be affected by primary preventive intervention is the workplace. No longer will employers and employees battle about issues of on-the-job safety. Employers will realize that safe work conditions are more economical than unsafe ones. Far fewer accidents and disease conditions such as black lung disease (pneumoconiosis) will originate in the occupational setting.

Each person will be provided with an individualized program of screenings, including physical examinations based on family history and other risk factors. Each individual will also assume responsibility for maintaining a health book containing a record of his or her physical examinations, immunizations, height, weight, allergies, illnesses, and accidents.

Health care providers will be both knowledgeable and humane. Their primary objective will be optimal care for clients, not economic or other personal gain. Because holistic care will be practiced rather than simply preached, iatrogenic problems will be almost nonexistent.

Facilities that provide health care will be found where they are needed, but regionalization will assure that costly duplication of equipment and personnel will be avoided.

With the articulation by the federal government of a health policy with a strong philosophical framework, research will no longer be disease-oriented and fragmented, but rather unified with a great deal of communication between researchers.

The ethical aspects of health care will be viewed as being as important as the technological aspects. No longer will the overriding questions of human rights in matters of life, death, and autonomy be subjugated to physical control by machines and inflexible institutional "rules." It will not be uncommon for hospitals to retain a consulting philosopher much as they might formerly have retained a consulting attorney.

Home care will be a common alternative for the terminally ill, for those with a chronic illness, and for the elderly. This will be accomplished under nursing auspices and community support systems, which will provide such necessities as meals and homemaking services, for example. Nursing homes and other long term facilities will have declined in number, but the quality of those remaining will be high. Hospices will be available for those who choose to die there and for the short term purpose of pain management or intense psychological support.

Day care for mentally ill persons will be more common than institutionalization. Clients will be hospitalized for a limited time when this is necessary, but "warehousing" people will no longer be practiced. Society will have acquired a more tolerant attitude toward those who behave in "peculiar" but harmless ways. Therapeutic sessions for clients and their families will be available.

Pregnant women will have several choices in regard to delivery: they may deliver their babies at home, at a birthing center, or in a hospital. Nurses and physicians will provide care. Nurse-midwives will handle uncomplicated deliveries and provide prenatal guidance and postpartum followup.

"Health care" will have replaced "medical care" as the term of choice. Professional care providers such as nurses, physicians, pharmacists, dietitians, social workers, and speech, occupational, and physical therapists will work together to provide optimal care. At times one health caregiver may be able to provide all the care. In other, more complicated situations, a team of people will be necessary. The choice of team leader will depend on the client's needs. The client will always be considered a member of the health team with the right to make the final decisions regarding care. No one will "own" the client.

We will have finally realized that prevention is more economical than cure and that prevention hurts less than cure—physically as well as economically. Cure will not be neglected, however. We will have a nationwide system of rescue vehicles staffed by highly trained paramedics. These vehicles and personnel will be in communication with emergency room personnel. A client who needs specialized care will be driven or flown to the nearest facility that can provide that care. When the illness or injury becomes less acute, the client will be returned to his or her community where care will be provided at a local hospital. This system will resemble the one presently used in the care of seriously ill neonates.

Health care givers will all receive the same basic educational preparation consisting of clinical courses and core studies in the sciences, including social science, before branching off into several broad fields. For example, one may prepare to become a provider of primary health care (traditionally the role of physicians and dentists), or a provider of care for the dishabilitated, or a health educator; or one may receive training in machine-related work involving diagnosis and treatment, or prepare for work in community organization, planning, or administration (1, pp. 197-198). In each area there will be both generalists and specialists. There will be no competition among professionals, only mutual respect. Individual professional organizations will exist primarily to certify schools and practitioners and to set standards. Interdisciplinary organizations will flourish as avenues for knowledge-sharing.

The structures of the professions will be markedly changed from those of today. No longer will women and minorities furnish the supporting base of the personpower pyramid. Rather than oppress a few so that those in the predominantly male occupations may reap even more power, prestige, and money, the pyramid will be a circle wherein each group is recognized for its expertise and each group gets a share of the pie, both in professional satisfaction and economic reward. "Nonprofessional" and "assistant" health care workers will be few in number and will be carefully chosen. They will find open doors for entering the health care discipline of their choice. Workers will be valued and committed to their jobs. Many fewer assistants will be needed than previously because professionals will be carefully utilized. Efficiency will be a high priority and will be achieved by the streamlining of paperwork and bureaucratic controls (27).

Current Trends in Health Care Delivery

Ethics

Interests in the ethics of health care has risen dramatically in recent years. It is not difficult to find the reasons for this upsurge of interest, which is overtly manifested by the increase in the numbers of ethics courses given in nursing and medical schools and the growth of such organizations as the Institute of Society, Ethics, and the Life Sciences, and the Hastings Center.

Barely a century ago, medicine had little to offer society. The science itself and the equipment available to it were primitive. Patients had hardly more than a 50 percent chance of being helped by medical intervention. As scientific and technological knowledge mushroomed during the twentieth century, the medical community found it had a great deal of power over life and death situations without a proportional gain in knowledge about ethical methods of handling that power. We have miracle medications and new methods of administering them; we have respirators that can breathe for a person and dialysis machines that can take the place of nonfunctioning kidneys; surgery is spectacular. We can bypass inadequate coronary arteries, reattach severed limbs, and cut out cancerous growths. With the use of ultrasonography we can "see" a baby while it is still in utero and, with fetal monitors, we can graphically see the fetal heartbeat during and between contractions.

Because this tremendous power over lives is a present reality, one needs to ask: *Who* should have the power and *what* decisions should be made?

Another reason for our increased concern about ethics is the issue of patients' rights. Consumers generally are now more informed about the products and services they are buying, and that includes health care. Because some researchers in the past blatantly ignored the human rights of their research subjects, the public demanded protection. As a result, the federal government has deveoped guidelines to protect research subjects.

Abortion, which had been illegal in this country since the latter part of the nineteenth century, is now legalized. This has engendered innumerable debates about when life begins and about fetal research.

One of the most vexing ethical problems facing health care providers and the public as the century draws to a close is the use of life-sustaining treatments. The President's Commission for the Study of Ethical Problems in Medicine and Biomedical and Behavioral Research deemed "the way decisions are and ought to be made about whether or not to forego life-sustaining treatment" important enough to warrant an investigation and the publication of a nearly 600-page book with the results of its inquiry (1a).

People are becoming concerned about the right of an individual to die a death unburdened by last-minute heroic efforts fraught with bodily invasion and pain, while often being deprived of the comfort of family and friends. In the interest of prolonging life, health care providers may scrimp on pain medication or place less importance on comfort measures than on the continuing use of high-technology equipment. The President's Commission reassured health care professionals that treatments that may risk death may still be used to relieve suffering as well as to promote a return to health (1a, p.73). As Ritchie said, ". . . . the theoretical right to be left alone fares poorly when confronted with the compulsion to use available life-prolonging technology" (1b). Slowly, changes are occurring even in the topics for debate. Professionals and lay people are openly discussing issues previously only whispered about. For example, the *Hastings Center Report* opened its pages to authors who argued various points of view about assisted suicide (1c, 1d).

The hospice movement exists so that those who are dying may find care and support rather than unwanted or unwarranted high technology intrusions.

Prevention

In the HHS publication *Prevention Profile,* five goals were set forth for 1990 (2). These are: to improve infant health by bringing down mortality by at least 35 percent to 9 per 1,000 live births; to improve the health and health habits of adolescents, lowering deaths between the ages of 15 to 24 by 20 percent to 93 per 100,000; to improve adult health by bringing down the death rate for that group by 25 percent or to 400 per 100,000; to improve older adult health by bringing the number of days of restricted activity down by 20 percent to less than 30 days per year for those 65 and older.

Modern technology comes with an expensive price tag. Therefore, society needs to make decisions about allocation of resources. This function has given rise to new ethical issues that deal with public policy and health, including the rationing of care (9). In addition, federal funds are utilized in so many areas of health care provision that financing health care becomes, *de facto,* the business of the national government.

Nurses are becoming more interested in the ethics of their professsion, and some are pursuing doctoral studies in that field. Nurses often find themselves in the center of ethical dilemmas with little knowledge or power to resolve the problems. Yet nurses are increasingly being held responsible for any omissions and commissions in their practice, whether they be inadvertent or intentional.

Health education is probably one of our most important weapons against disease and accidents, and there are some signs that this concept is taking hold. Some states mandate that school systems include health education in their curriculums. Professional organizations such as the American Dental Association and the American Medical Association sponsor television advertisements with health education themes. Other groups, including the American Cancer Society, promote anti-smoking campaigns. At least one study has shown that individual health behavior is unpredictable; consequently the highest level of success in changing behavior seems to come from attacking specific problems such as smoking, diet, and inactivity rather than from trying to improve health behaviors in a more general way (3, p. 1144). There is much work and research to be done in health education,but as the above examples indicate, governmental and private groups are beginning to show a respect for this concept and its potential impact for good on the health of the nation.

One cannot discuss prevention without mentioning the importance to society of maintaining the health of women and children, including such preventive activities as counseling, amniocentesis to detect genital defects, rubella vaccination (5; 6; 7; 8), prenatal, intrapartal, and postpartal care, good childhood nutrition, immunizations, and mental health programs.

Although many women in the United States receive prenatal care, substantial numbers do not. In 1988, changes in Medicaid eligibility were proposed to ensure care to more pregnant women and their infants. Although the evidence is incomplete, there appears to be a relationship between no prenatal care and the incidence of higher-risk, low birth-weight infants. Readers particularly interested in barriers to and access to prenatal care will want to read an American Nurses' Association publication (10).

A recently published study showed that access to health insurance for poor women does not ensure that they will get prenatal care nor that pregnancy outcomes will be improved. The researchers speculated that the reasons might be that some providers refuse to care for poor women because of lower reimbursement rates and increased paperwork. They also speculated that policies toward women's health that were more broadly articulated so that women would enter pregnancy in better health might have secondary positive effects on infant outcome. In addition, factors other than health care have influences on health outcomes. Issues of poverty, housing, nutrition, and education must be addressed (10a).

In the utopian health care system described earlier in this chapter, industrial safety was identified as an important part of the national effort to promote accident and disease prevention. There are encouraging signs that safety in the workplace is becoming the goal of both employers and employees. One example is the coal mining industry. Even though coal mining continues to be the most dangerous of occupations, there has been a significant decline in fatalities among miners over the past decade. The Coal Operators Association and the coal workers' union have made a series of joint statements on safety which represent a model of cooperation between employers and employees. These two groups also sponsor training programs for workers whose job is to monitor safety in the mines (11).

As the century draws to a close, the nation is gathering ideas for healthy goals for the year 2000 (12). Since resources are finite, we are already faced with rationing of care. But we spend more per capita on health care than virtually any other country (9). Is a focus on prevention one way to get more for our health dollars?

Health Care Institutions

Because of multiple factors, among them the skyrocketing costs of hospitalization, home health care would seem to be a viable, cost-effective alternative. Prospective payment schemes for hospitalization have placed sicker persons back into the community and forced us to reexamine home health care as an alternative. The Health Care Financing Administration, the overseer of Medicare and Medicaid, has announced interest in projects to demonstrate what home care agencies can do in terms of quality of care and cost-effectiveness. Nurses are the best prepared professionals to provide leadership in home care (13).

Another trend concerns childbearing. Although there are some areas of the country where home births have always been the norm, in most areas during the past half century the hospital has become the place where women go to have babies. Now we seem to have come full circle. Home births are becoming increasingly popular. Although many health care professionals do not advocate home births, others support the concept. One physician shares his thoughts about home births thusly: "Professional assistance is necessary and emergency procedures should be readily available. I'm not against hospital deliveries; it's just that surgery is overutilized and the vital human considerations are largely ignored" (15).

Another fairly recent phenomenon is the childbirth center. It exists outside the hospital environment and offers prenatal, intrapartal, and postpartal care. These centers, which are adaptations of the home setting, provide safe care to families during a normal childbirth experience. Stringent criteria are used to screen clients. Even so, the centers usually are equipped for emergencies. They have facilities for administering oxygen, blood volume expanders, and emergency drugs. They have resuscitation equipment, a neonatal transport circulator, and a system for ambulance transfer, if necessary, to a back-up hospital. The members of the staff include obstetricians, certified nurse-midwives, pediatricians, public health nurses, and support personnel. Clients are usually discharged within 12 hours of delivery. A public health nurse visits the family within 24 hours and again a few days later. Telephone consultation with a caregiver is always available (16, p. 755).

In-hospital birth centers, often called birthing rooms, are appearing in many places. Featured are home-like rooms where labor and delivery take place. Usually the woman is free to assume the position most comfortable for her. Continuous or electronic fetal monitoring is usually not part of the service. Some families opt for early discharge while other women may spend a few days in the postpartum unit. Many hospitals are modernizing their maternity units by combining labor, delivery, recovery, and postpartum rooms so that a woman remains in the same private room from admission to discharge. These are known as LDRP rooms.

Regionalization

Sharing expensive facilities and equipment by people in a circumscribed geographic region is becoming an important means of cutting the costs of health care. Milio says that in some states which had received federal construction grants, 35 to 40 percent of hospital beds were unused (1, p. 90). The extensive development of costly equipment and machines for diagnosis and cure has often resulted in competition among hospitals instead of cooperation. In too many instances expensive machinery has stood idle.

Regionalization also capitalizes on the the expertise of personnel. Hospitals that do 20 open-heart operations in a month, for instance, have more qualified personnel than hospitals that do one such operation per month. Nurses and physicians who work in neonatal intensive care units become more expert in their field than those on the staff at a hospital that consistently has a small neonatal census.

One detriment to regionalization is that the patient's family may have difficulty in getting transportation to the larger, specialized facility. However, very often, as soon as the patient has improved, he or she is returned to the community hospital, particularly when the patient is an infant. Treatment for many cancer patients is begun and regulated at a metropolitan center and then the responsibility for care is transferred to the home community as soon as possible.

The National Health Planning and Resources Development Act of 1974 (see Chapter 3), even though not using the word "regionalization," makes provisions for its implementation. Some objectives of the act are to control the number of underused and unused facilities, to help correct the maldistribution of health care facilities and workers, and to have the decisions about expenditures for new construction made at the local level. Additionally, it provides for primary care services for the underserved, the coordination of or consolidation of institutional health services, the development of multi-institutional arrangements for sharing special services necessary to all health service institutions.

We are moving in the right direction. Time will tell whether or not we as a society are committed to the concept of regionalization.

Nurses as Care Providers

The following discussion will focus on two roles for nurses, neither one new, but rather resurging. The first is the role of nurse-midwife, the second, that of nurse practitioner. (See Chapter 6 for an in-depth discussion of health care providers.)

The last decade has seen a marked increase in the number of midwives. Even though midwives had been the principal birth attendants throughout history, they were systematically stripped of their roles by the nineteenth century. Midwives were not allowed the "privileges" of using operative obstetrics as were male physicians, nor were they admitted to schools where they could learn obstetrical techniques. Midwives hesitated to use procedures such as version of the fetus because they feared being branded as witches if the woman or fetus were to die (17).

In the United States, the status of midwives reached its peak during early colonial times. Then, as medicine became increasingly professionalized, midwives were increasingly discredited (18). It was not until 1931 that the New York Maternity Center Association's school for midwives opened. Eventually, other schools opened and, by 1973, 1,400 midwives delivered about one percent of the babies born in the United States. Midwives deliver 80 percent of the babies in the rest of the world.

Beginning in 1965, nurse practitioners have now approximately a quarter century of experience and are making major contributions to health care (4). Nurse practitioners are often described as practicing in an "expanded role." Educational preparation for this role is often provided in a university setting although not necessarily attached to a degree-granting program. These nurses learn skills such as history taking and physical assessment. Some states require that they be certified in order to practice as practitioners. Certification examinations are given under the auspices of such groups as the American Nurses' Association, The American College of Nurse Midwives, and the Nurses' Association of the American College of Obstetricians and Gynecologists.

Preparing for the Role of Nurse in the Twenty-First Century

A Delphi survey of fellows of the American Academy of Nursing generated a list of ten items of importance to the profession. These might be considered as an agenda for nursing in preparation for practice in the twenty-first century. Foremost among the items are the public image of nursing, developing public awareness of the unique contribution of nursing to health care, and creating public acceptance of nursing as an independent profession (24, pp. 8-9).

There is dissension in the house of nursing as to the roles nurses are to play in the decades to comes. If nurses practice nursing, their role is complementary to that of physicians and other health care professionals. If they purport to be physician substitutes, then they are rightfully fearful for their jobs and physicians are justified in feeling threatened. Nursing and medicine will overlap at times, but each profession has unique expertise to offer clients. Four items from the Academy's Delphi survey relate to clarifying nursing in the public view as an independent profession with unique services to offer. These are: 1) conducting research nationwide on the cost of nursing services delivered in nursing models; 2) ensuring the autonomy of nursing through nursing practice acts; 3) promoting the role of private third party payers for nursing services; and 4) establishing nurses as the primary providers in hospice care (24, p. 9).

If we in nursing can speak as one voice for better health care, perhaps we can make a positive impact on the health care delivery system. We need to prepare nurses who are sophisticated in planning, in policy making, and in influencing political processes. Health care consumers are important allies for nursing. We must let the public know what we can do (19, pp. 4, 6). We must develop a cadre of nurses who have effective skills in the political arena (24, 1981, p. 9, 25).

An important way for nurses who work in institutions to use their intellectual and creative abilities while being accountable for the nursing care they provide is through primary nursing. Primary nursing helps to ensure that clients know who their nurses are and begin to develop an understanding of how nurses can meet many of their health care needs. The time seems ripe for the acceptance of a philosophy of nursing that uses the skills of the professional nurse for the improvement of care, increases the nurse's level of satisfaction, encourages clinical research, and supports collegiality with other professionals (20, p. 68). McClure et al.'s 1983 magnet hospital study (26) highlights the creation of climates in hospitals that foster nursing practice at its best. The strategies and programs of the institutions in the sample are important to the future of nursing practice and deserve careful study and replication. These hospitals exemplify one issue raised in the Delphi study cited earlier—to "ensure a control of [the] work setting that enables real nursing to be practiced and taught" (24, p. 9).

Recently there has been much discussion and disagreement about the "entry into practice" issue. Although nursing has a long history of university education for its members beginning with the University of Minnesota's program in 1909, nurses with degrees are still in the minority. In 1965, the American Nurses' Association took the position that there should be two separate and distinct educational programs in nursing and two categories of nursing practice—essentially, technical and professional. The Association, in 1978, reaffirmed its earlier stand.

Since the mid-nineteen sixties many diploma schools of nursing have been phased out. However, the confusing multiplicity of educational programs preparing people for licensure as registered nurses still exists. The licensure exam is still the same for the graduates of all of these programs. Small wonder that we in nursing have had difficulty explaining our roles to the consumers of health care.

How Can Nurses Influence Change?

That nurses must practice their clinical skills in a knowledgeable, humane, and ethical way would probably not be disputed by many nurses or the public. What is not as clear to many nurses and the public is that nurses need a more global awareness than the microcosm of their practice arenas in order to effect change for public health and practice issues. One of the most powerful ways for nurses to count as a unified voice is through membership in the American Nurses Association (ANA). As the largest group of health care professionals, nurses collectively have the potential to influence change. As individuals, nurses can help to influence local and state legislation by keeping abreast of legislative proposals and testifying for or against these proposals at public hearings. There are many examples of how the professional association works on behalf of improved health care.

The nursing profession, through the ANA, was included in the transition cluster group by the Clinton administration. The purpose of the group was to evaluate the Department of Health and Human Services. As her representative in the group, the President of the ANA, Virginia Trotter Betts, appointed Myra Snyder, RN, deputy major for health and human services for the city and county of San Francisco (28). The voice of nursing was also heard at a meeting of the Task Force on National Health Care Reform on March 3, 1993. The Task Force's Chair, Hillary Rodham Clinton, expressed agreement with the ANA philosophy as set forth in *Nursing's Agenda for Health Care Reform (see Chapter 3 for an outline of the agenda),* especially concerning the issues of removal of anti-competitiveness barriers which prevent nurse practitioners, clinical nurse specialists, and nurse midwives from practicing to their full potential (27, 29). On May 6, 1992, nurses rallied in Washington, D.C. for health care reform. *The American Nurse* said, "The rally is just one example of nurses' increased political activism during 1992 and the profession's grass-roots efforts across the U.S." (29).

As this book goes to press, the nation awaits the announcement from the White House about the direction of health care reform. It is exciting that nurses are being included in the process. Twelve nurses are members of a panel of 47 professionals who will critique proposals of the Health Care Task Force (30). Whether proposed legislation is national in scope or originates at the state or local level, nurses need to be able to analyze it. To that end, the Massachusetts Nurses Association developed a flyer entitled "Moral Dimensions of Public Policy Formation: Guidelines for Nurses" (see Chapter 3). The document addresses issues of respect for persons; the health, welfare, and safety of the client; and the distribution of social benefits and social burdens. Its purpose is to assist nurses to evaluate proposed legislation and policies.

Other resources that nurses have at their disposal are research studies and their own experiences based on clinical practice. For example, to show that nurses could be a partial solution to the health care crisis, the ANA used the results of a study that found nurse practitioners provided primary care that was as good as or better than the care provided by physicians (31).

Self-Care and Self-Help

Self-care implies that a layperson maintains his or her own health. People have always cared for themselves but there is more organization for this among the laity now. Levin's description of the values of self-care sound as though they would fit beautifully into our concept of the ideal health care system. These values are "human integrity, freedom of choice and action, achievement of health status as the layperson sees it, and self-fulfillment and happiness" (21, p.210).

The current self-help movement, which has its roots in feminism, is a response to what was perceived as inadequate, often sexist,and inhumane care. Feminist groups met to share and research information. For instance, they used vaginal specula to visualize their cervixes in order to discover early changes that might indicate a health problem. Many of these groups developed into women's clinics which have a unique philosophy of care. There are no barriers between clients and caregivers; clients are truly partners in their own care.

Health care professionals have often clashed with self-help groups. This is unfortunate because of a phenomenon which occurs when women become involved in learning about their bodies. That is, they begin to see the relationship between good health habits and their own health. The health care system must learn from the consumers what their needs are and incorporate suggestions so that we no longer alienate those we claim to serve.

Summary

Many of the trends in health care delivery are headed in the right direction. As citizens and as taxpayers, consumers will ultimately have the final say on the shape of the health care system. This is an exciting time; many novel programs are being tried and are succeeding. The next two decades may well be the most critical ones of this century in shaping the course of health care in the year 2000. Technological advances, the knowledge explosion, escalating costs, the political and legislative climate, consumer power, and the refocusing on ethics and human rights of the past two decades have laid a foundation for the future. Upon this foundation we can build a utopia, replicate the present structure, or create a slum. As the most numerous professional providers in the system, nurses can be major architects for health care circa 2000 A.D.

References

1. Milio, N. (1975). The Care of Health in Communities: Access for Outcasts. New York: Macmillan.
1a. President's Commission for the Study of Ethical Problems in Medicine and Biomedical and Behavioral Research. (1983). Deciding to Forego Life-Sustaining Treatment. Washington, DC: U.S. Government Printing Office.
1b. Ritchie, K.S. (1990). The last remaining way to die. Hastings Center Report 20(3):2-3.
1c. Nicholson, R.H. (1993). A quick and painless death. Hastings Center Report 23(3):5.
1d. Kamisar, Y. (1993). Are laws against assisted suicide unconstitutional? Hastings Center Report 23(3):32-4l.
2. United States Department of Health and Human Services, Public Health Service. (1983). Prevention Profile. Washington, DC: United States Office of Disease Prevention and Health Promotion, pp. 243-246.
3. Mechanic, D. (1979). The stability of health and illness behavior: Results from a 16-year follow-up. American Journal of Public Health 69:1142-1145.
4. Henry, O.M. (1986). How many nurse practitioners are enough? American Journal of Public Health 76(5):493.
5. Krugman, S. (1979). Rubella immunization: Progress, problems and potential solutions. American Journal of Public Health 69:217-219.
6. McLaughlin, M.C. and Gold, L.H. (1979). The New York rubella incident: A case for changing hospital policy regarding rubella testing. American Journal of Public Health 69:287-289.
7. Falvo, C.F., Weiss, K.E., and Liss, S.M. (1979). A rubella screening and immunization program in an adolescent clinic. American Journal of Public Health 69:283-285.
8. Chappell, J.A. and Taylor, M.A.H. (1979). Implications of rubella susceptibility in young adults. American Journal of Public Health 69:279-281.
9. Lamm, R.D. (1986). Rationing of health care. The Nurse Practitioner 11(5):57,61-62,64.
10. Curry, M.A. (1987). Access to Prenatal Care: Key to Preventing Low Birthweight. Kansas City: American Nurses Association.
10a Hass, J.S. Udvarhelyi, S., Morris, C., and Epstein, A.M. (1993). The effect of providing health coverage to poor uninsured pregnant women

in Massachusetts. Journal of American Medical Association 269:87-91.

11. Franklin, B.A. (1980, Nov. 27). New effort to make mines safer. The New York Times, p. 29.

12. Now for health objectives after 1990. (1988). The Nation's Health 18(7):12.

13. Rinke, L.T. (1987). Replacing a failing old pattern with a vital new paradigm. Home care. Nursing and Health Care 8(6):331-333.

14. Osterweis, M. and Champagne, D.S. (1979). The U.S. hospice movement: Issues in development. American Journal of Public Health 69:492-496.

15. Sorenson, P. (1976). Birth at home. Synapse, April 29, p. 1.

16. Lubic, R.W. and Ernst, E.K.M. (1978). The childbearing center: An alternative to conventional care. Nursing Outlook 26:754-760.

17. Corea, G. (1977). The Hidden Malpractice: How American Medicine Treats Women as Patients and Professionals. New York: Morrow, p. 221.

18. Walsh, M.R. (1977). Doctors Wanted: No Women Need Apply. New Haven: Yale University Press, p. 5.

19. Stanhope, M. (1979). Politics: The Nurse and the Health Care Consumer. New York: National League for Nursing, Pub. No. 41-1778), pp. 4,6.

20. Clifford, J.C. The potential of primary nursing. In: Health Care in the 1980s. Who Provides? Who Plans? Who Pays? New York: National League for Nursing, Pub. No. 52-1755, p. 68.

21. Levin, L. (1976). The layperson as the primary health care practitioner. Public Health Reports 91:206-210.

22. Kibrick, A.K. (1981). Accountability, review boards, and the lay participant. Nursing and health Care 2(3):124-129.

23. Nursing in the year 2000. (1984). Image 16(1):entire issue.

24. Lindeman, C.A. (1981). Priorities Within the Health Care System: A Delphi Survey. Kansas City, MO: American Academy of Nursing.

25. Rains, J.W. (1988). Nursing and politics: Adapting skills to spark social change. Nursing and Health Care 9(6):299-301.

26. McClure, M.L., Poulin, M.A., Sovie, M.D. and Wendalt, M.A. (1983). Magnet Hospitals. Kansas City, MO: American Nurses Association.

27. Nursing's Agenda for Health Care Reform. (1991). Washington, DC: American Nurses Association.

28. Nursing represented on Clinton transition team. (1993). The American Nurse 25(1):1.

29. Hillary Clinton seeks nursing's input on reform. (1993). The American Nurse 25(4):1-2.

30. Nurses to critique Clinton health plan. (1993). American Journal of Nursing 93:72.

31. Study shows nurse practitioner care may rival physician primary care. (1993). The American Nurse 25(2):3.

Index

LONGMAN LINGUISTICS LIBRARY

VERB AND NOUN NUMBER IN ENGLISH: A FUNCTIONAL EXPLANATION